Priority Setting Toolkit:
A guide to the use of economics in healthcare decision making

D0981086

To Michelle and Diane

Priority Setting Toolkit: A guide to the use of economics in healthcare decision making

Craig Mitton

Centre for Healthcare Innovation and Improvement, BC Research Institute for Children's and Women's Health and Department of Health Care and Epidemiology, University of British Columbia, Vancouver, Canada

Cam Donaldson

Center for Health Services Research, School of Population & Health Sciences and Business School (Economics), University of Newcastle upon Tyne, Newcastle upon Tyne, UK

© BMJ Publishing Group 2004
BMJ Books is an imprint of the BMJ Publishing Group

First published in 2004
by BMJ Books, BMA House, Tavistock Square,
London WC1H 9JR

www.bmjbooks.com

British Library Cataloguing in Publication Data

A catalogue record for this book is available from the British Library

ISBN 0 7279 1736 6

Typeset by SIVA Math Setters, Chennai, India
Printed and bound in Spain by GraphyCems, Navarra

Contents

Preface

Around the globe, healthcare systems, and health organisations within those systems, are faced with a common dilemma. As resources are limited, choices have to be made about what services to fund and what not to fund. Choices must also be made about the extent to which services will or will not be funded. No additional influx of resources will alleviate the fundamental need to make these choices. The reason is simple: the needs and wants in health care will always outstrip the resources available.

This challenging task of making choices in health care is complicated by any number of factors, including the following:

- limited training for decision makers in economic and ethical concepts
- a lack of understanding of formal approaches to priority setting
- limited information to support trade-offs
- a diverse set of stakeholders and the competing values of those groups
- the often non-rational behaviour of organisations.

This book seeks to provide a clear, non-technical depiction of the economic concepts underlying priority setting in health care, and through this, to present a specific way forward for explicit, evidence-based priority setting for application by decision makers in health organisations. Challenges to this activity, and specific means of overcoming these challenges, are also outlined.

Much of the practical information contained in the Toolkit stems from our experiences with priority setting over the last 15 years, in Britain, Australia and Canada. We are thus indebted to the many colleagues, both fellow researchers and decision makers alike, with whom we have worked over this time and who have advanced our understanding, particularly in the "how to" of this challenging topic.

We offer our heartfelt thanks to Joan McGregor, Stephen Singleton and Roy Mitton for taking the time to critically review the book and provide many helpful comments. We would also like to thank Diane Lorenzetti for her assistance with updating the literature in Chapter 6, and to acknowledge with gratitude the support of Mary Banks and Christina Karaviotis from BMJ Books.

We also thank Elsevier Science Ltd for granting permission to reproduce Figures 5.1 and 6.3, Blackwell Publishing for permission to reproduce Table 4.1, and the CD Howe Institute, Toronto, Canada, for permission to use material for parts of Chapter 2 including Figure 2.1.

The Canadian Health Services Research Foundation provided salary support to Craig Mitton in the form of a post-doctoral fellowship during the time the book was written. Craig Mitton took up this award (2001–2003) in the Calgary Health Region, the Centre for Health and Policy Studies, University of Calgary, Alberta, Canada, and the Division of Health Sciences, Curtin University, Perth, Australia. Cam Donaldson holds the Health Foundation Chair in Health Economics and is an ESRC Advanced Institute of Management Research Public Services Fellow (2003–4).

Craig Mitton
Cam Donaldson

Part 1: Background

1: Introduction

The priority setting challenge

In most countries, health care is managed and administered by health organisations that have the responsibility to meet, as best they can within a limited funding envelope, the health needs of a pre-defined population.* This worldwide phenomenon has been brought into focus by various healthcare reforms and other system-level developments, and has resulted in local decision makers being required to set priorities and allocate resources.

In the UK, such an arrangement has existed for over half a century, with health authorities managing and administering the system in the form of the National Health Service (NHS). Recently, the need for local decision making was reaffirmed through the establishment, in England and Wales, of primary care trusts which have responsibility for commissioning services in line with the needs of their local populations.[1] Similar arrangements, involving a commissioner or purchaser of services having to function with limited funding, have been put in place, or are currently being considered, throughout western Europe.[2-6]

In eastern Europe, an important reform in Russia was the transfer of budgetary responsibility to polyclinics, which bought services on behalf of their patients.[7] Since that time, such reforms have struggled to get off the ground, but attempts to mirror them in other eastern European countries have been tried by giving financial responsibility to arms-length intermediaries.[8]

In South American countries, there has also been a growing use of such intermediaries. In Argentina, Chile and Columbia,

---

*Note that the term "health organisation" is used generically to represent any body which is allocated a fixed amount of money on a regular basis (usually annually) to plan health service provision for a pre-defined population. The covered population could be defined geographically, such as in the cases of health authorities, health boards, health regions, health districts, and primary care trusts, or through prepaid enrolment, such as in the case of health maintenance organisations or other managed care organisations.

intermediaries have been encouraged to compete more with each other to attract enrolees and, in turn, to encourage competition amongst providers.[9-11] Whilst the increased enrolment of large numbers of poor people has been cited as a key achievement of these publicly funded systems, a series of constraints undermining access has been identified.[11] In any case, these developments have left decision makers to set priorities at the local level.

In other countries, such ideas are newer. For example, in Canada the very notion of "regionalisation" (which does not go as far as independently functioning purchasers and providers or the use of an arms-length intermediary) is a mid-1990s phenomenon in most provinces, and includes legislated mandates to health authorities for priority setting.[12] Even in the USA, the move to managed care in the 1990s has brought the need to set healthcare priorities into sharper focus.[13,14]

Despite a mix of Commonwealth and State healthcare funding in Australia, where there has been a system of integrated health organisations since 1984, local bodies must make choices about what to fund and what not to fund. Finally, New Zealand, which has one of the oldest public healthcare systems in the world, experimented throughout the 1990s with various forms of organisational and funding models.[15]

All such health organisations face a common challenge. As there are more claims on resources than there are resources available, some form of priority setting must occur.[16] That is, resources are scarce and there is thus a need, regardless of how many resources are available in total, to make choices about what to fund and what not to fund. This may be in the form of commissioning services, as is done in the UK and elsewhere, or in dividing up a pool of resources within regional health authorities, as is the case, for example, in Canada and Australia.

Recent work, however, has suggested that decision makers within health organisations may require assistance with priority setting.[17,18] In addition, the allocation of resources in health organisations tends to be conducted on the basis of historical patterns, but this can lead to suboptimal use of the limited resources available. In fact, it is clear, at least in some jurisdictions, that measuring the "return on investment" and planning for how resources should best be spent are not always very far advanced.[19] What is required, and indeed what decision makers seem to be asking for, is a systematic, explicit approach to priority setting which is fair and, where possible, evidence based.

In today's climate, with strong economic pressures facing every society, the relevance of priority setting is clear. Where to cut, where to expand, and how to conduct these processes are critical questions. As well, there are also a number of wider challenges to priority setting in health care which have to be taken into account, such as the extent of public participation in the process, whose values are to be used at what level of priority setting, what would a *fair* process for priority setting look like, and how should technical judgements of the clinical professions be married with the value judgements of those charged with allocating the resources. In addition, in certain jurisdictions, local decision makers must respond to recommendations from national level bodies, such as the National Institute of Clinical Excellence (NICE) in England and the National Health Committee in New Zealand. While these bodies are concerned about quality across the board, national recommendations must be met locally, leaving decision makers having to make trade-offs under yet more constraints than might otherwise have been the case.

A major question, then, becomes whether there is a process for priority setting which responds practically to the dilemma of resource scarcity. Such a process should be conducted in a manner which is as evidence based as possible and, at the same time, must also encompass a large range of wider challenges, as referred to above.

Two economic concepts

As economics is generally viewed as "the science of choice", it is proposed that this discipline can help to guide healthcare decision makers in using resources in the best manner possible. Two important economic concepts which are referred to throughout this book are opportunity cost and the margin. The former emerges directly from the recognition that resources are scarce, and, as such, choices invariably have to be made. With resources always being limited, by choosing to implement one option, there is a benefit forgone as resources

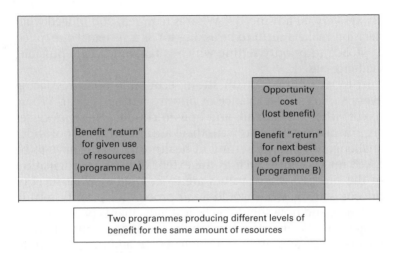

Benefit "return"
for given use
of resources
(programme A)

Opportunity
cost
(lost benefit)

Benefit "return"
for next best
use of resources
(programme B)

Two programmes producing different levels of
benefit for the same amount of resources

Figure 1.1   Illustration of opportunity cost

are then not available for other options. The lost benefit from
the next best use of the resources is the opportunity cost.
Referring to Figure 1.1, other things being equal, a decision
maker would, hopefully, allocate resources to A in preference
to B. Although some benefit is lost by not investing in B, this
is less than would be the case if A were sacrificed instead.

An important goal that can be reached through priority
setting activity is to maximise benefits and, conversely,
minimise opportunity costs. The logical implication of
applying this concept is that one needs to know both the
resources used as well as the health and other gains obtained
from various healthcare options. It is this information which
allows decision makers to optimally deploy limited healthcare
resources.

Thanks to the second concept mentioned above – the
margin – one does not have to measure the costs and benefits
of all new and existing healthcare options on an ongoing
basis. The margin has to do with the benefit gained or lost
from adding or subtracting the next unit of resources for a
given programme. The size of the programmes does not
matter; it is the gains (or losses) that are realised by putting
more resources into (or taking resources away from) each
programme at the margin that is the key. For the programmes

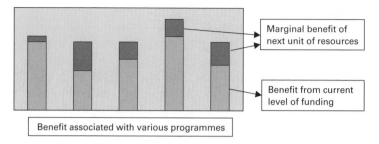

Figure 1.2 Marginal benefit of next unit of resources

illustrated in Figure 1.2, if each programme were to be expanded by one unit of resources, the programme second from the left would be the preferred choice, again all things being equal, as the greatest marginal benefit is realised for this programme.

So, in a given healthcare setting, if one extra dollar were to be made available, that dollar should ideally be invested in the area in which the most benefit (however defined) will be gained in return. Conversely, if the budget in a given setting was to be contracted by one dollar, the first dollar to be taken out should, in theory, be obtained from the area where the least benefit will be lost. Furthermore, even in a stable funding situation, thinking at the margin enables decision makers to consider shifting or *re*allocating resources in a manner which will improve patient benefit overall.

The importance of the margin stems from the fact that it is about changing situations in such a way as to make them better. Increasing benefits from limited healthcare resources is what being efficient, or being more efficient, is all about. Two different types of efficiency which are central to healthcare priority setting are outlined in Chapter 2. As other important goals are of course sought through priority setting activity, such as improving equity (or fairness), the focus throughout the book is not only on maximising benefits from limited resources but more broadly is about using resources in a manner in which various locally defined criteria, or principles, are best met.

The Toolkit

To address the issues raised above, this book seeks to provide decision makers with a set of tools to put the economic concepts of opportunity cost and the margin into practice within health organisations. Recognising the complexity of real world decision making, the challenge is to do so in a pragmatic enough manner so as to provide a practical aid for decision makers. As no one "gold standard" for priority setting stands out in the literature to date, a number of approaches to priority setting are initially outlined, with comparisons enabling critical appraisal in relation to the economic concepts mentioned above.

In the end, what will be seen as the way forward has more to do with a way of thinking about the economic concepts, and the consequent principles of efficiency and equity, than with a single approach for setting priorities. Part of the Toolkit, therefore, involves being aware of the concepts which underlie an economics-based approach to priority setting. That said, and coming back to the practicalities, one particularly useful approach to priority setting which permits these economic concepts to be operationalised is programme budgeting and marginal analysis (PBMA). It is this approach, which has been used in health organisations over the past three decades, that forms the basis of this Toolkit.

Despite the positive impact of PBMA in many areas, challenges remain in its implementation, providing an explanation for why even greater use has not occurred. The approach itself, case studies to exemplify its application and a number of challenges related to PBMA and other explicit approaches to priority setting are presented in this book. It is also useful to recognise early on that having an explicit approach for priority setting is only part of the solution. While the primary focus of the Toolkit is on the "how to", it is also recognised that there is a need to evaluate the process of priority setting itself.[14] Drawing the "how to" and the "evaluation" together is considered herein.

Overview of this book

The overall purpose of this book is to provide practical guidelines for healthcare priority setting and, as well, an in depth understanding of related issues, for managers, clinicians and health researchers. In this way, the book offers a set of tools to carry out priority setting, and also intends to stimulate debate and challenge the way of thinking for all those interested in or charged with the difficult task of setting healthcare priorities.

The specific aims of this book are:

1 To outline the basic concepts of an economic approach to healthcare priority setting.
2 To appraise critically several approaches to priority setting, out of which one, PBMA, will be put forth as the most useful way forward.
3 To provide a detailed set of steps for carrying out a PBMA process and an inventory of activities to date in the use of PBMA.
4 To demonstrate, through the use of case studies, how economic concepts can be put into practice at different levels in health care.
5 To highlight specific challenges in moving from theory to practical and useful applications which can make a difference in the real world of healthcare delivery.

While the focus of this book, as illustrated in the sub-title ("the use of economics in healthcare decision making"), is on the contribution of health economics to priority setting in health organisations, the information in the book has clearly benefited from contributions from other disciplines. Although it is emphasised that any priority setting framework used in health care should adhere to the economic concepts of opportunity cost and the margin, these concepts on their own are not enough. This is illustrated by the fact that economic approaches to priority setting, despite having been shown to be useful in specific contexts in the past, have not to date generated universal appeal.

As will be uncovered in the following chapters, it is only through collaborative efforts between the various stakeholders including patients, clinicians, managers, ethicists, organisational behaviourists, health economists and health services researchers that a comprehensive approach to priority setting can result, as shown in Figure 1.3. In the end, these different streams are brought together in the hope of offering a launching pad not only for those making decisions to move

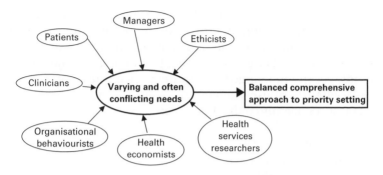

Figure 1.3 Stakeholder relationship and basic objective

forward with the important task of priority setting, but also for researchers to join together in future collaborative efforts.

The book opens with a detailed discussion of the two fundamental economic concepts, already outlined in brief above, along with two key principles in health care, efficiency and equity. Following this, in Chapters 3 and 4, a number of widely used approaches to healthcare priority setting are critically appraised against these economic concepts, and an ethical framework that is currently gaining some recognition is presented as a means to evaluate priority setting activity.

In Chapter 5, the PBMA process is presented in a practical, step by step manner. A detailed description of the history of PBMA and its use internationally, including its impact, is then provided in Chapter 6. In order to illustrate the use of PBMA, case studies from Britain and Canada are presented in Chapter 7. In so doing, it will be demonstrated that PBMA, and, as such, an economic way of thinking, can be used to inform priority setting at different levels within health organisations.

As alluded to, numerous challenges to explicit, evidence-based priority setting activity exist, and some of these are highlighted in Chapters 8 through 12. These chapters serve as a response to a number of matters raised in the literature relating not only to PBMA, but also to other explicit, evidence-based approaches to priority setting. Importantly, none of these challenges would seem to be insurmountable for forward thinking decision makers willing to stand up to the political forces and "do the right thing".

The book closes with an outline of next steps for moving the priority setting agenda forward, in both the real world of decision making and the land of academia. While it is intended that managers and clinicians will have a much better handle on the practical doing of priority setting after reading the Toolkit, it is also thought that, more generally, progress depends on decision makers and researchers working together.

Summary

In summary, the following are some of the key points addressed throughout the book.

- The devolution of responsibility for management and delivery of health services in most countries has led to the need for local decision makers to set priorities and allocate resources.
- Whatever the amount of resources received for health care, some means of priority setting is required to divide up the available resources amongst the competing claims.
- There is scope for helping managers and clinicians to gain a better understanding of approaches to priority setting and thereby advance decision making beyond historical patterns of allocation.
- The economic concepts of opportunity cost and the margin should underpin any approach for setting priorities, but these in and of themselves are not enough.
- PBMA operationalises the economic concepts in a pragmatic and useful manner, and serves as the basis for the "way forward" presented in this book.
- As can be expected, numerous challenges to explicit priority setting in healthcare organisations exist, although none would seem insurmountable.
- Various academic disciplines must work together with decision makers to inform the way forward for priority setting in health care.

The formation, in 1996, of the International Society for Priorities in Health Care implies not only that priority setting in health care is now globally recognised but also that there is a desire to share experiences of the many priority setting practices which exist in different jurisdictions. The time is now to "make a start" and, to paraphrase Voltaire, "to not let the best be the enemy of the good". While there is still much work to be done in priority setting in health care, significant and exciting strides in this area have been made in the past decade. Although "the best" may not yet have been reached, it is hoped that this Toolkit can serve as an important step in moving forward.

References

1   NHS Department of Health. *Corporate governance framework manual for primary care trusts.* www.doh.gov.uk/pct/2002/corpgovframeworkmanualaug02.doc (accessed 29 Jul 2003).
2   Van de Ven WMM. *A future for competitive health care in the Netherlands.* NHS White Paper Series, Occasional Paper No. 9. York: Centre for Health Economics, University of York, 1989.
3   Hakansson S. New ways of financing and organizing health care in Sweden. *Int J Health Plann Manage* 1994;9:103–24.
4   Linna M. Health care financing reform and the productivity change in Finnish hospitals. *J Health Care Finance* 2000;26:83–100.
5   Segouin C, Thayer C. The French prescription for health care reform. *Int J Health Plann Manage* 1999;14:313–27.
6   European Observatory on Health Care Systems. *Health Care Systems in Eight Countries: Trends and Challenges.* London: London School of Economics and Political Science, 2002.
7   Hankansson S, Majnoni d'Intignano B, Roberts J, Zollner H. *The Leningrad Experiment in Health Care Management 1988. Report of a visit to the USSR.* Copenhagen: World Health Organization, 1988.
8   Ensor T, Thompson R. Health insurance as a catalyst to change in former communist countries? *Health Policy* 1998;43:203–18.
9   Hsiao W. Colombia health system reform. *AHSR and FHSR Annual Meeting Abstract Book* 1995;12:120–1.
10   Jack W. *Health Insurance Reform in Four Latin American Countries. Theory and Practice.* Policy Research Working Paper 2492. Washington DC: The World Bank Development Research Group, Public Economics, 2000.
11   Plaza B, Barona A, Hearst N. Managed competition for the poor or poorly managed competition? Lessons from the Colombian health reform experience. *Health Policy Plann* 2001;16 (Suppl 2):44–51.
12   Province of Alberta. *Regional Health Authorities Act: Chapter R-9.07.* Edmonton: Queen's Printer for Alberta, 1994.
13   Freund D, Hurley R. Medicaid managed care: contribution to issues of health reform. *Annu Rev Public Health* 1995;16:473–95.
14   Daniels N, Sabin J. The ethics of accountability in managed care reform. *Health Affairs* 1998;17:50–64.
15   Ashton T, Cumming J, Devlin N. Priority-setting in New Zealand: translating principles into practice. *J Health Serv Res Policy* 2000;5:170–5.
16   Birch S. Making the problem fit the solution: evidence based decision making and "dolly" economics. In: Donaldson C, Mugford M, Vale L. eds. *Evidence Based Health Economics: From Effectiveness to Efficiency in Systematic Review.* London: BMJ Books, 2002.

17 Lomas J, Woods J, Veenstra G. Devolving authority for health care in Canada's provinces: 1. An introduction to the issues. *Can Med Assoc J* 1997;**156**:371–7.
18 Mitton C, Donaldson C. Setting priorities in Canadian regional health authorities: a survey of key decision makers. *Health Policy* 2002;**60**:39–58.
19 Donaldson C, Mitton C, Currie G. *Managing Medicare: the Prerequisite to Spending or Reform.* The Health Papers No. 157. Toronto: CD Howe Institute, 2002.

2: Economic concepts

Introduction

The central notion in this chapter is that no matter how many resources are available in total, the focus should be on how best to deploy those resources. The chapter opens with three reasons why attention needs to be paid to managing, as compared to simply expanding, the available resources. Two economic concepts, introduced briefly in Chapter 1, are then addressed more fully, along with their consequent implications for efficiency and equity. This health economics grounding is important at an early stage in developing the Toolkit, as it is these concepts and principles that are the foundations on which the priority setting discussions are based in each of the following chapters. Before closing, the economic concepts are illustrated with both real and hypothetical examples.

More resources or better management?*

Scarcity is here to stay

The first and most striking reason for not solely relying on more resources for health care is that scarcity is here to stay, and thus must be dealt with no matter the size of the healthcare budget.[1] That is, the claims on resources for health services will always be greater than the resources available. Therefore good management of the currently available resources is required, whereby lower priority items are traded off for more highly valued items. While this rationale may seem simplistic, it has stood the test of time and points directly to the need to examine how best to allocate the current pot of resources.

---

*Parts of this section, including Figure 2.1, are taken from: Donaldson C, Mitton C, Currie G. *Managing Medicare: the Prerequisite to Spending or Reform*. The Health Papers No. 157. Toronto: CD Howe Institute, 2002.

Improving health

Second, if an objective of government is to improve health, the payoff may be higher by injecting more tax dollars into better housing or education rather than health care. This is because healthcare spending is not the only input into the production of better health, and in fact may have quite a small impact relative to other factors.[2] As is well known, broader social determinants such as housing, education, diet, lifestyle and the environment all influence health.[3] Given that there may be other ways in which health can be improved, the main question becomes whether extra money allocated towards these other determinants could lead to greater improvements in health than spending on health care.

In fact, research from over thirty years ago found that education had more potential for reducing mortality than did an increase in per capita health spending.[4] Others have also found that higher income and schooling have positive effects on health as well as access to health care,[5] and it has been argued that past improvements in mortality in developed countries have owed more to environmental factors (for example hygiene and sanitation) than to medical care.[6] Marmot suggests that social, economic and political factors all have an important influence on health and longevity.[7] Thus, why should the focus continue to be on increasing spending on *health care*? Instead, it could be argued that the main concern should be in dividing up the limited health resources available amongst health care and other sectors of the economy that contribute to health. Of course, this line of thinking may well mean that all healthcare "needs" are *not* met.

For each dollar put in, what comes out?

Third, the issue just outlined can be examined through considering more explicitly the return obtained through investing more resources in health care. Figure 2.1 shows the hypothetical relationship between benefits and healthcare spending, holding all other determinants of health constant. The level of spending on the horizontal axis could be interpreted, for example, as total national spending. Whether

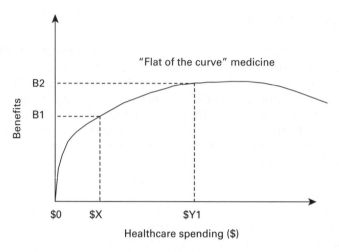

Figure 2.1 The effects of increased healthcare spending

more should be spent on health care depends on the *additional* health benefits gained from spending on health care compared with the *additional* benefits gained from spending the same amount on some other sector that contributes to health, such as education. When examined, it may be that at levels of healthcare expenditure between zero and $X the extra benefits from increased healthcare spending are greater than those from using the same resources elsewhere. In such a situation, more should be spent on health care.

There will come a point, however, where the extra benefits achieved by greater healthcare spending will be less than the benefits of diverting that spending elsewhere. In the diagram, this could be beyond the point where $X are spent. It may be that health is generated by putting resources into other sectors of the economy (or other healthcare treatments). If so, $X should be the maximum spent on health care. If spending is increased beyond this point, up to $Y for example, then more benefits are forgone than are produced and society is worse off. At $Y, with benefits of B2, maximum benefits are being generated on the "flat of the curve". Any extra spending is unproductive in terms of extra health gains. If more and more continues to be spent then eventually total benefits could decline and patients may be harmed. The problem is that it is not clear whereabouts on this curve we lie. Indeed, the whereabouts may vary depending on the viewpoint of a specific stakeholder (see Figure 1.3).

There is much evidence of "flat of the curve" practice from the USA. For example, rates of inappropriate surgery for carotid endarterectomy range from 13 to 32%.[8-10] For tonsillectomy and coronary artery bypass surgery, rates of inappropriate surgery have been estimated to be 86% and 14%, respectively.[11,12] In Canada, such variations have been observed in various kinds of surgery both within and between provinces.[13,14] As variations in practice exist, governments and the public may ask why they should invest more in the healthcare system.

Dealing with scarcity: the basis of economics

Regardless of whether more resources are added to the healthcare pot, there is a need for an explicit and informed approach to the allocation of current and future healthcare resources. Even if the decision maker or politician, in the end, wants to advocate for expanding the pot of resources for health care, it is the case that at some point decisions must be made about how best to spend the resources that are available. If healthcare decision makers want to obtain the best out of what amounts at any point in time to a limited budget, economics can be used to assist this process. Two key economic concepts, and a decision matrix which emerges from these concepts, are considered here.

Opportunity costs

Economics and priority setting go hand in hand. Each is based on the undeniable fact that resources are scarce. Choices thus have to be made about what services to provide and what not to provide. No matter what worthy statements are made about rights of access to care, some rights will be met while others will not, or at least, not immediately. How then can decisions be made about where resources should be spent?

The basis of the economic response to this question is the concept of opportunity cost. In the context of having to make choices within the constraint of limited resources, certain opportunities will be taken up while others must be forgone. The benefits associated with forgone opportunities are opportunity costs. If the aim is to maximise benefits to the community – and conversely minimise opportunity costs – there is a need to measure the costs and benefits of health care. "Costs" here reflect resources used, as it is in using resources that opportunity costs arise. "Benefits" represent gains in health and well-being brought about by the use of resources. By measuring costs and benefits, the deployment of resources which maximises benefits from available resources can be chosen.

Marginal analysis

The task of measuring costs and benefits should be done through marginal analysis. This involves starting with a particular mix of services and analysing changes in that mix. If resources can be shifted to produce greater benefit then this should be done. Such changes are often not about whether to introduce or eliminate a service in totality but rather are about whether to have more of one service or less of another. Regardless of how many resources are available, examining changes at the margin enables benefit to be increased *for the given budget.*

If a focus on health gain is taken, for example, this goal is reached when no further reallocation of resources from one service to another will result in an increase of total benefit.[15] In theory, this is the point where the ratio of marginal costs to marginal benefits across services is equal. How to identify this optimal point is discussed below. Marginal analysis is concerned with the last unit of production of any two or more given programmes; the best mix of services is determined by examining the relative costs and benefits of the various options, *at the margin.* This type of analysis highlights trade-offs, which can help decision makers to weigh up proposals for change on the basis of the marginal costs and benefits of the given options.

Failure to adopt these economic concepts will mean that maximal health gain (assuming "health" is a goal) is unlikely to be reached. That is, in deciding to allocate resources towards a particular programme, or in making a decision to treat a given patient, an often implicit decision is being made not to provide some other service or treatment. If no explicit consideration is given to the lost benefits of not funding the alternative services, it is then less likely that benefit overall will be maximised. While the discussion here has focused on benefit as in "health gain", the points can also be extended to a broader set of outcomes, as highlighted below. It is also worth mentioning that these comments focus on the provision of services; clearly not everyone who has capacity to benefit will seek out or have access to relevant care options.

A decision matrix *

How can information on costs and benefits be used to help make decisions? A simple framework is proposed, based on two forms of efficiency which arise from the concepts of opportunity cost and marginal analysis. The starting point is to consider that all health organisations currently deploy resources in some way or other. Any change in the way care is delivered is likely to have an impact on both health outcomes and costs. By first deriving and second linking estimates of relative costs and outcomes of alternative procedures under consideration, it should be possible to determine whether replacing current care with some new procedure results in:

- higher costs and better outcome than current care, in which case a judgement would have to be made about whether the extra cost is worth the gains in health achieved. (This is an "allocative efficiency" question, as treating the same number of patients by some different option will mean using more resources for this group and having fewer available for another group)
- lower costs and the same or better outcome as current care, in which case the change would be judged to be a better use of healthcare resources (i.e. more "technically efficient").

While these two forms of efficiency (i.e. technical and allocative) are discussed in more detail later, it is the case that

*Parts of this section are taken from: Donaldson C, Mitton C, Currie G. *Managing Medicare: the Prerequisite to Spending or Reform.* The Health Papers No. 157. Toronto: CD Howe Institute, 2002.

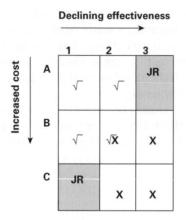

Declining effectiveness

√, yes/adopt; X, no/reject; √X̄, indifferent;   JR, judgement required

Outcome

Compared with the control treatment, the new treatment has:

1. evidence of greater outcome
2. evidence of no difference in outcome
3. evidence of less outcome.

Cost

Compared with the control treatment, the new treatment has:

A. evidence of cost savings
B. evidence of no difference in costs
C. evidence of greater costs.

Figure 2.2 Matrix linking effectiveness with cost. Adapted from the Cochrane Collaboration. *Cochrane Collaboration Handbook.*[16]

in any context information on outcomes and costs can be summarised in a matrix format to aid in the judgement about whether a new procedure is preferable to the current situation. As per Figure 2.2, adapted from the *Cochrane Collaboration Handbook*,[16] it can be seen that, relative to the status quo, a new procedure could achieve a greater outcome, the same level of outcome or less outcome. In terms of cost, a new procedure could save costs, result in no difference in costs or increase costs.

For any procedure, where a new treatment is in cell A1 of the matrix, i.e. it would both save costs and have greater health outcomes relative to current care, then it is clearly superior to current care. In fact, in cells A1, A2 and B1, the new procedure is more efficient than current care and is assigned a √ in response to the question of whether it is to be preferred to current care. In cells B3, C2, and C3 the new procedure is less efficient than current care and thus receives a X response. In cells A3 and C1 a judgement would be required as to whether extra health benefits justify the extra costs (C1) or the cost savings justify the lost benefits (A3).

For example, in cell C1 there is a cost involved, in the sense that the extra resources required to implement the new procedure would have to come from some other group of patients. In both A3 and C1, economics can highlight the magnitudes of extra resources required and outcomes gained. There is however, a judgment required beyond that as to whether the extra benefits might justify the extra costs involved. Finally, cell B2 is neutral, as there is no difference in either costs or effectiveness. As will be seen in Chapter 4, the programme budgeting and marginal analysis (PBMA) approach can operationalise this decision matrix and thus provides decision makers with a tangible means of weighing service options in regard to both technical and allocative efficiency.

Two key aims: efficiency and equity

Efficiency

Now that the economic concepts underlying resource allocation in health care have been examined, two of the main aims in health care are briefly examined: having an efficient system and having an equitable system. The first of these, efficiency, has already been introduced but a more detailed explanation is provided here.

Broadly speaking, efficiency can be defined as maximising well-being at the least cost to society. In fact, efficiency is intimately related to opportunity cost. As already alluded to, a goal in health care is likely to be to maximise benefit with the resources available. The closer society is to achieving this goal, the more efficient the healthcare system will be. If there is an inefficient use of resources, the allocation could be changed in some manner to realise increased health benefits, or, more broadly speaking, well-being. Through marginal analysis, potential changes in the mix of services provided for a given budget can be highlighted to identify how the efficiency of the programme might be increased.

As mentioned, there are two specific types of efficiency to keep in mind in reading the rest of the Toolkit. First, allocative efficiency relates to whether or not something is worth doing given its opportunity cost. In the healthcare context, this type of efficiency is reached if no greater benefit can be provided from some other mix of services for the given resources. When decisions about changes in resource use are made at this level, one group of patients will benefit at the expense of another. The trade-off arises because, within a fixed budget, to fund more of one service less funding must be implicitly or explicitly put towards another service. If resources were not scarce, all claims on resources could be met through the funding of all services required or desired. Once it is accepted that resources are scarce, however, it follows that choices over the claims on resources must be made. With priority setting across programmes, a goal is to arrive at a mix of services which maximises benefit for the given resources. The closer the healthcare system is to this point, the more allocatively efficient it will be.

The second type of efficiency is technical or operational efficiency. This type of efficiency asks the question: What is the least cost manner in which to obtain a particular objective? In terms of health care, for the same group of patients, a choice would be made between different treatment options. In other words, given that a health services programme has already been allocated some resources, the question is, "In what manner should these resources be spent so that the benefit is maximised?". Alternatively, it could be said that if two treatments provide the same benefit, the more technically efficient option would be the treatment that is less costly. Strictly, improved technical efficiency is about increasing the output – for example the health benefit – for a given set of inputs or producing the same level of output with less of one input and more of others.

In the following chapters, it will become apparent that the PBMA approach can deal with concerns pertaining to both allocative and technical efficiency. Prior to examining a number of practical scenarios, the notion of equity is first discussed.

Equity

Given scarcity, it can be argued that the distribution of resources should not only follow a pattern which produces the most benefit overall, but should also be fair. Equity is about fairness. It is often the case, however, that there is a conflict or trade-off required between efficiency and equity. For example, centralisation of services geographically may well increase efficiency but may make access for those in rural areas disadvantaged in comparison with those in the cities. The value healthcare decision makers place on the principles of efficiency and equity may vary across contexts and societies. It is thus important for decision makers to determine the criteria on which priority setting decisions are to be made as well as the relative weights to be attached to these criteria.

More specifically, equity can be considered in terms of horizontal and vertical equity. Horizontal equity refers to the "equal treatment of equals" while vertical equity refers to the "unequal (but equitable) treatment of unequals".[17] The point here is not to enter a lengthy debate on how best to define equity, but rather to point out that it is important for decision makers to define the criteria upon which allocation decisions will ultimately be made, and to make those definitions explicit. Nonetheless, drawing on previous work by Mooney,[17] a number of definitions of equity can be offered, as shown in Box 2.1. While equality of health may be next to impossible, it could be a preferred working definition in certain contexts where the aim, say, is to raise the level of health of disadvantaged groups, through a disproportionate allocation of the pot of resources available.

Box 2.1 Potential definitions of equity

- Equality of expenditure per capita
- Equality of inputs per capita
- Equality of inputs for equal need
- Equality of access for equal need
- Equality of utilisation for equal need
- Equality of marginal met need
- Equality of health

Once the criteria are determined and defined, shifting of resources at the margin can lead to getting the most out of those resources, whether that be in terms of maximising benefit (i.e. improving efficiency) or moving towards equality of health (i.e. improving equity). A further important issue has to do with ranking or weighting the criteria, as in all likelihood, at some level, a choice will have to be made between degrees of efficiency and degrees of equity. It is thus useful for decision makers to determine:

1 the relevant criteria for priority setting
2 definitions for these criteria
3 a hierarchy, or preferably, relative weighting, of the criteria.

Illustrating the concepts: real and hypothetical case studies

Marginal analysis of one programme

To illustrate these concepts, economists often refer to what has become something of a classic in health economics, the case of the sixth stool guaiac.[18] In the mid-1970s, the American Cancer Society recommended that, when attempting to detect asymptomatic cancer of the colon, an individual's stool sample be tested six times. The first part of a sample would be tested, and, if positive, the subject would have further confirmatory tests and treatment as required. If negative, the second part would be tested. If positive, the subject would have further confirmatory testing and, if negative, the third part would be tested, and so on. A screened person would be declared negative only after all six parts had tested so. Neuhauser and Lewicki's analysis of this policy showed that about 66 of the expected 72 cases, or 92%, are detected after the first round of testing, at a cost of US$1175 per case detected (Table 2.1). The second round of testing ensures most cases (99.2%) are detected at an average cost of US$1507 per case. Six rounds capture almost all cases (99.9%) at a cost per case of US$2451.

Another way to look at these same data, however, is in terms of the *extra* costs and *extra* cases detected from each successive round of testing (Table 2.2). In other words, what are the

Table 2.1 Cases detected (from a population of 10 000) and costs of screening with six sequential tests

No. of tests	Total cases detected	Total costs (US$)	Average costs (US$)
1	65·9469	77 511	1175
2	71·4424	107 690	1507
3	71·9003	130 199	1811
4	71·9385	148 116	2059
5	71·9417	163 141	2268
6	71·9420	176 331	2451

Table 2.2 Marginal benefits (cases detected) and marginal costs of successive screening tests for cancer of the colon

No. of tests	Marginal benefits* (cases detected)	Marginal costs (US$)*	Ratio of marginal costs to marginal benefit[†]
1	65·9469	77 511	1175
2	5·4956	30 179	5492
3	0·4580	22 509	49 150
4	0·0382	17 917	469 534
5	0·0032	15 024	4 724 695
6	0·0003	13 190	47 107 214

*Here the term "marginal" refers to each successive round of screening rather than one more person screened.
[†]Variation due to rounding.

marginal costs and marginal benefits? The second round detects an extra 5.5 cases compared with one round, with the extra cost being US$30 179, or US$5492 per case. Round six over round five provides little extra gain, at an extra cost per extra case detected of over US$47 million! As can be seen, this example is definitely in cell C1 of the matrix in Figure 2.2.

Referring back to the theoretical concepts of opportunity cost and the margin, the US$47 million indicates that the opportunity cost of the $13 190 spent on having six rounds rather than five is probably too great. The reason is that these resources could most likely produce more benefit elsewhere. In a cash-limited healthcare system, the screening of the colon service "at the margin" would be reduced and the resources re-invested elsewhere, producing more benefits overall. The

Table 2.3 Marginal benefits and marginal costs of two sub-programmes

| | Sub-programme A | | | | Sub-programme B | | | |
Unit	Marginal costs $	Total costs $	Marginal benefits $	Total benefits $	Marginal costs $	Total costs $	Marginal benefits $	Total benefits $
1st	10	10	35	35	20	20	60	60
2nd	10	20	30	65	20	40	50	110
3rd	10	30	25	90	**20**	**60**	**40**	**150**
4th	**10**	**40**	**20**	**110**	20	80	30	180
5th	10	50	15	125	20	100	20	200
6th	10	60	10	135	20	120	10	210
7th	10	70	5	140	20	140	0	210
8th	10	80	0	140	20	160	0	210

implication of this is that the data on costs and benefits for one programme against those of another programme must be compared. To illustrate this, two more examples, one hypothetical and one real, are provided.

Marginal analysis of two programmes

An example first developed by Mooney et al.[15] involves a decision on what balance of resources to allocate between two sub-programmes within a programme of care. In Table 2.3, for sub-programme A, the marginal cost of each successive additional unit is assumed to be constant (i.e. $10). Thus, total costs rise in increments of $10 as more and more units are produced. For programme B, the marginal cost is $20, and so the total costs rise in $20 increments.

A further assumption is that the benefits of each sub-programme, such as health gain, can be valued in monetary units. Two points need to be emphasised here. First, there clearly are difficulties in measuring benefits in the same units as costs. This is done here merely for ease of exposition and to illustrate economics as a "way of thinking" about priority setting. Second, note that the benefits of each sub-programme in this example are assumed to decline as more and more of the programme is provided. This is reasonable in that one could imagine that those patients with more to gain get

Table 2.4 Combinations of sub-programmes within the budget constraint

Sub-programme A		Sub-programme B		Total programme (A + B)	
Units	Benefit $	Units	Benefit $	Total benefit $	Total cost $
8	140	1	60	200	100
6	135	2	110	245	100
4	**110**	**3**	**150**	**260**	**100**
2	65	4	180	245	100
0	0	5	200	200	100

treated first. This assumption of declining marginal benefit is crucially important to the mechanism of marginal analysis.

Taking each sub-programme in isolation, a decision maker would not provide A beyond six units because, beyond this point, the benefit gained from having one more unit is less than the cost of providing that unit. So, the service should be provided up to the point where marginal benefits are equal to marginal costs. Likewise, with sub-programme B, five units would be provided. Beyond six units of A and five of B, the resources involved in producing additional units could be better spent elsewhere. In other words, the opportunity cost of these resources would be too great if used to further expand A or B.

Now assume that, for the programme overall, there is a fixed budget constraint of $100. What is the optimal level of provision of A and B? In Table 2.4, it can be seen that, if provision is heavily weighted towards A, such as having eight units of A and only one of B (thus exhausting the $100 budget), total benefit will be $200. Having six of A and two of B is better, producing $245 worth of benefits (remembering that this represents health gain and other sources of well-being). At the other extreme, the whole budget could be spent on five units of B, thus producing $200 in benefits.

The benefit-maximising position, however, is four units of A and three units of B, producing $260 worth of benefits. Looking back at Table 2.3, an important thing to note about these levels of provision, highlighted in bold, is that their ratios of marginal benefit to marginal cost (20/10 for A and 40/20 for B) are equivalent, i.e. each ratio equals 2, whilst the total budget is also exhausted. Referring back to the subsection above on marginal analysis, the point where these ratios are equal provides the signal that no more switching of resources between sub-programmes A and B can increase total benefit.

Marginal analysis of several programmes

Still, a number of questions remain, such as:

- How can these concepts be operationalised, given that costs and benefits usually cannot be measured in the same units?
- Can more than just two programmes be compared?

The notion that is introduced here, and is picked up again later in the Toolkit, is that of resource *re*allocation. That is, in order to have the preferred allocation of resources, however defined, some shifting of resources from one programme to another will be required. As such, resources can be disinvested in one area and re-invested elsewhere. In a priority setting exercise conducted in Canada, a healthcare manager came up with the following example in an attempt to explain the process to his colleagues.

First, assume that there will be $12 million of service development monies coming into the health organisation in the next financial year. The organisation, therefore, after having established some criteria to allow for comparison, such as "health gain", "contribution to national priorities", etc., has come up with the list of priorities displayed in Table 2.5 (a). It can be seen from the table that only the first four proposals can go ahead for development as, when combined, they take up the whole of the $12 million (hence the dotted line under the fourth proposal).

Second, assume that, amongst the senior managers who have compiled the rankings, there is considerable support for items further down the list – items a5 through a10. This means that, if the organisation is to fund any of these further proposed developments, it must consider reducing costs, and perhaps levels of service, elsewhere. Therefore, corresponding to the prioritised list of service developments, a list of areas for release of resources would have to be compiled, as in Table 2.5 (b).

Table 2.5 Costs (and cost savings) from service developments and areas of resource release

	Programme	Cost (savings)
(a) Service developments	a1	$4 m
	a2	$2 m
	a3	$3 m
	a4	$3 m
- -	a5	$2 m
— · — · — · — · — · — · — · — · — · — · — · — · — · — · —	a6	$1 m
	a7	$1 m
	a8	$4 m
	a9	$0·5 m
	a10	$3 m
(b) Areas of resource release	b1	($0·5 m)
	b2	($1·5 m)
— · — · — · — · — · — · — · — · — · — · — · — · — · — · —	b3	($1 m)
	b4	($4 m)
	b5	($2 m)

- - - - - - - - - - - up to here, developments are paid for from "new money"
— · — · — · — · — up to here, $2 m is taken out of b1 and b2 and put into a5
———————— up to here, $1 m is taken out of b3 and put into a6

Assume that the first two of these result in no loss of benefits to patients as they are the result of technical efficiency improvements. So, the same level of service can be provided with fewer resources, remembering cells A1, A2 and B1 in the decision matrix in Figure 2.2. This allows one more programme to be funded, hence the second dotted line in Table 2.5 (a). To go further down the list in Table 2.5 (b) would result in some loss of benefit in other areas and would require the management group to compare the benefits lost through "cuts" with the gains to be had by shifting these resources into the remaining options in (a).

Assume that the group decides that it is worth switching resources to option a6 by cutting or scaling back one more programme in (b), i.e. b3. After that, when the fourth programme in Table 2.5 (b) was compared with service development item a7, and part of a8, it was decided that it was better to stay with the status quo, hence the positioning of the solid lines in the table.

This process, which did not involve actually having to measure everything in the same units, is still based on the same concepts or "way of thinking" underlying the earlier examples. In Table 2.5 (a) and (b), a judgement has been made that there is no point continuing reallocations beyond the levels indicated by the solid lines because, *in toto*, nothing would be gained. Also, it should be noted that although there has been no explicit mention of equity in these examples, some explicit equity criterion, or criteria, could have been used when deciding on the ordering of developments and releases and, therefore, in deciding how far down to go in each list. Thus, in this respect, although they are often seen as separate issues, equity and efficiency can also be construed as part of one overall concept of well-being.

Summary

The need for rationing is not new, and can be summed up by stating that no matter how many resources are available in total, choices must be made between competing claims on the limited resources. At whatever level, it is important to bear in mind that the question is not usually whether to provide a service, but rather *how much* of it to provide. Ham[19] has observed that health organisations have "avoided excluding services entirely from their contracts". This view is not too far removed from the economics perspective which says that rationing is about having more of some services and less of others, rather than introducing or eliminating whole services. Once the idea of the margin comes into play then listing and de-listing of entire services ceases to be a rational way of expressing priorities.

Furthermore, decision makers may not always go for the "ideal" service at least from a clinical perspective. This was shown in the sixth stool guaiac example (see Table 2.1), as it may not be worth detecting every case of cancer that is out there. Strides towards maximising benefit across healthcare services will be made only when costs and benefits of various options are explicitly weighed. Through identifying opportunity costs, decision makers can then, for example, take resources from the last stage of screening cancer and invest elsewhere to achieve greater health gain. As many decision makers in health care may already be making intuitive decisions at the margin, what is being advanced here is that this type of healthcare decision making becomes more explicit and systematic.

From empirical analyses, Klein and Redmayne have observed that many UK health organisations are comfortable with no explicit rationing at all.[20] Such a desire to avoid explicit rationing is not surprising but it is likely to lead to lower efficiency and less equity than would otherwise be the case. Part of developing an explicit process for priority setting is making clear the criteria, and relative weighting of the criteria, on which priority setting decisions will be based. As will be discussed in Chapter 3, there is also a need to evaluate the priority setting process itself.

In this chapter, the basic components of a toolkit were outlined to get to the point of making priority setting decisions more explicit and systematic. Like many tools in a toolbox, it will be seen, particularly in Chapter 4, that they may not always be used precisely in the ways intended. They remain essential however, to achieving maximal benefit, or better meeting other important criteria, from limited healthcare resources. The basic components are:

- opportunity cost
- marginal analysis
- a decision matrix based on concepts of allocative and technical efficiency
- equity.

Prior to turning to an explicit approach for managing limited resources based on opportunity cost, marginal analysis and the decision matrix, a number of other approaches are first reviewed in Chapters 3 and 4. In the end, the approach put forth as the way forward attempts to make healthcare priority setting more explicit and formalised but also seeks to recognise that health organisation decision makers work in extremely complex environments, hence the need for pragmatism, but a pragmatism based on sound principles which allow scarcity to be managed.

References

1 Birch S. Making the problem fit the solution: evidence based decision making and "dolly" economics. In: Donaldson C, Mugford M, Vale L, eds. *Evidence Based Health Economics: From Effectiveness to Efficiency in Systematic Review*. London: BMJ Books, 2002.

2 Filmer D, Pritchett L. The impact of public spending on health: does money matter? *Soc Sci Med* 1999;**49**:1309–23.

3 Evans RG, Barer ML, Marmor T, eds. *Why Are Some People Healthy and Others Not? The Determinants of Health of Populations*. New York: Aldine De Gruyter, 1994.

4 Auster R. The production of health: an exploratory study. In: Fuchs VR, ed. *Essays in the Economics of Health and Medical Care*. New York: Columbia University Press, 1972.

5 Corman H, Grossman M. Determinants of neonatal morbidity rates in the US: a reduced form model. *J Health Economics* 1985;**4**:213–36.

6 McKeown T. *The Role of Medicine: Dream, Mirage or Nemesis? 2nd edn.* Oxford: Basil Blackwell, 1979.

7 Marmot M. Social determinants of health: from observation to policy. *Med J Aust* 2000;**172**:379–82.

8 Merrick NJ, Brook RH, Fink A, Solomon DH. Use of carotid endarterectomy in five California veterans administration medical centers. *JAMA* 1986;**256**:2531–5.

9 Chessin MR, Kosecoff J, Winslow CM *et al.* Does inappropriate use explain geographic variations in the use of health services? *JAMA* 1987;**258**:2533–7.

10 Winslow CM, Solom DH, Chassin MR *et al.* The appropriateness of carotid endarterectomy. *N Engl J Med* 1988;**318**:721–7.

11 Roos NO, Roos LL, Henteleff PD. Elective surgical rates – do higher rates mean lower standards? *N Engl J Med* 1977;**297**:360–5.

12 Winslow CM, Kosecoff JB, Chassin M, Kanouse DE, Brook RH. The appropriateness of performing coronary artery bypass surgery. *JAMA* 1988;**260**:505–9.

13 Gentleman J, Vayda E, Parsons G, Walsh M. Surgical rates in subprovincial areas across Canada: rankings of 39 procedures in order of variation. *Can J Surg* 1996;**39**:361–7.

14 Hartford K, Roos L, Walld R. Regional variations in angiography, coronary artery bypass surgery, and percutaneous transluminal coronary angioplasty in Manitoba, 1987 to 1992: the funnel effect. *Med Care* 1998;**36**:1022–32.

15 Mooney G, Russell E, Weir R. *Choices for health care: a practical introduction to the economics of health provision*. London: Macmillan, 1986.

16 Cochrane Collaboration. *Cochrane Collaboration Handbook*. Oxford: The Cochrane Collaboration, 1995.

17 Mooney G. *Economics, medicine and Health Care, 2nd edn.* Brighton: Wheatsheaf, 1992.

18 Neuhauser D, Lewicki AM. What do we gain from the sixth stool guaiac? *N Engl J Med* 1975;**293**:255–8.

19 Ham C. Priority setting in the NHS: reports from six districts. *BMJ* 1993;**307**:435–8.

20 Klein R, Redmayne S. *Fair shares for all?* NAHAT Research Paper No. 11. Birmingham: National Association of Health Authorities and Trusts, 1993.

Part 2: Approaches to priority setting

3: "Non-economic" approaches to priority setting

Introduction

In many countries, local managers and clinicians have been given responsibility to set health priorities and allocate resources accordingly. While tools have been suggested to aid this process, both knowledge of these tools within health organisations and comparative analysis in the literature are limited. This chapter, along with Chapter 4, summarises the state of the art of some of the most common approaches to priority setting, on the basis of their adherence to the economic concepts presented in Chapter 2 and as well on their impact in practice to date. Three "non-economic" approaches are described and appraised in this chapter.

- Historical allocation and decibels
- Needs assessment, including burden of disease, and the related approach of cost-of-illness
- Defining core services.

As will be seen, these approaches ignore the fundamental concepts of opportunity cost and the margin, and thus when employed, benefit maximisation will not be achieved. As such, they are not best used for the purposes of setting priorities in health care.

The Accountability for Reasonableness framework is also introduced in this chapter as a means of evaluating priority setting activity. The focus with this framework is not so much on the resulting decisions of priority setting, but rather on how well the process itself stands up to a number of relevant ethical conditions.

In Chapter 4, several "economic" approaches to priority setting are examined, which are based on the key concepts presented in Chapter 2. As will be demonstrated, however, even economic approaches, in their application, can at times ignore opportunity cost and the margin. Thus, decision makers should be aware of potential pitfalls when using the various approaches for priority setting. In the end, a particular economic method will be promoted, which can also work with or encompass some of the other approaches reviewed, such as the Accountability for Reasonableness framework, discussed below, and economic evaluation, discussed in Chapter 4. Prior to addressing the above mentioned approaches to priority setting, however, a number of characteristics for priority setting approaches, identified from the literature, are outlined.

Characteristics

Given the economic concepts introduced in Chapter 2, a prerequisite for a priority setting approach is the ability to consider questions of equity as well as efficiency.[1,2] A review of the literature also indicates that a priority setting process should be open and explicit[1,3–6] and that involvement of the public is preferable.[1,7–9] It is also held that evidence from research should play some part in the decision making process,[10,11] and that national priorities should be incorporated.[1,2] It is also suggested that the process should be based on an ethical framework.[8] In short, the required characteristics are demanding, challenging and complex.

Of course, in any given context, a particular approach to priority setting may have some of these characteristics and not others. In the end, the important point is that the process is fair; the above characteristics will likely contribute to this, and as mentioned, more formal tools to evaluate this are available. Further, even if some "ideal" is not met, as Cohen[12] states, it is "improvement that is sought, not perfection". Any approach should be compared to current practice, and in so doing, it should be asked whether or not the processes of priority setting have been improved. These characteristics, along with the economic concepts of opportunity cost and the margin, can be kept in mind as the approaches themselves are considered.

Current practice in priority setting

As highlighted in Chapter 1, responsibility for setting priorities and allocating resources has been devolved to the local or regional level in many countries. While the specific decision making process in any given health organisation will likely vary, some formal work has been done to describe priority setting activity in various contexts. For example, a survey of over 60 senior managers in three health regions in Alberta, Canada, provided insight into the processes at work.[13] This survey found that, at the time, no formal process of setting priorities and allocating resources existed in the three regions. That is, the respective processes were largely ad hoc, with little consideration given to issues of transparency and explicitness. Allocations were made based on historical trends, with some adjustments made each year for demographics or political will. In the sample, the majority of respondents stated that the process of allocating resources across programmes did not work well. Key suggestions for improvement from the group included the implementation of an explicit, systematic approach to priority setting and improved communication between administrators and physicians.

This reflects experience in the UK in the 1990s, during the time of the internal market. For example, survey work by Miller[14] and Vale[15] indicates that historical allocation processes were at play in England and Scotland, and again that managers were looking for more informed, explicit processes for setting priorities and allocating resources. Which decision makers are to be charged with making which decisions was also observed to be important. The reality of political influence has also been observed in priority setting exercises in Australia.[16] It is within these contexts that the various priority setting "tools" can be set.

Common approaches to priority setting

Historical allocation and decibels

As alluded to, the most common approach to priority setting and subsequent resource allocation in health organisations is to base funding decisions on what has been funded traditionally. As such, in actuality no formal approach to priority setting is followed. This historical allocation process can be made more elaborate to greater or lesser degrees with the inclusion of adjustment factors to account for changes in health service costs or the population base. Another term for such priority setting is "what you got last year plus a little more or less, depending on the budgetary situation". As a lack of explicit priority setting activity is endemic within this type of approach, it is common for local politics to enter into the process. This latter mechanism could be known as the "decibel approach".

Importantly, neither history nor decibels provide a mechanism for maximising health benefit within a given budget.[17,18] The reason is that they fail to recognise the underlying concepts of opportunity cost and the margin. In addition, practically speaking, managers and clinicians find little satisfaction with these approaches,[13] as politics and implicit values rather than sound judgement and transparent decision making take control of the organisation's priority setting processes. It is not clear why funding in these manners is so common, but one could imagine that in the reactive culture of most health (and indeed in many other) organisations they take the least amount of time to implement. Although it should be noted that there may be inherent value in the status quo, in the UK at least there has been a call to challenge these inherited patterns of priorities, in particular across programmes within the health organisations.[19]

Needs assessment

Needs assessment is a commonly used tool in priority setting. One approach to needs assessment is to define need either at the individual or population level, and then set a minimum standard of care (or set of services) to meet that need. "Need" can be defined by whether or not a treatable condition exists, and then evaluative techniques can be used to measure the met and unmet needs of the particular population based on this definition.

Defining need in this way is challenging however because need is value based, and the values taken are often those of a third party rather than the patient. It is thus dependent on who that third party is. For example, a clinician may feel that an individual has a need – for example, a man's prostate is enlarged – but the individual may choose to ignore his symptoms, decide that there is no "need" at all and not "demand" treatment. Further, attempting to set a minimum standard, such as six rounds of testing to screen for cancer, ignores the reality that there may not be enough resources available to meet this minimum standard, and thus some sort of priority setting is still required.

Another concern is that needs assessments seldom consider explicitly the resource impact of implementing priorities on the basis of the needs assessment estimates. Thus, while attempts may be made to change the mix of services provided based on the met and unmet needs of the population, no consideration is being given to the costs of doing so. This would mean that priorities might not change if, say because of some technological advance, extra heart transplants were able to be conducted at half their previous cost. Further, priority setting is about how best to use resources to intervene in providing health and other benefits. Therefore, it is interventions or policies that should be prioritised as they are what consume resources. Identifying unmet need may help to identify where a potential gap in services exists, but does not inform about how much resources should be spent in that area.

A second form of needs assessment is an epidemiological or burden of disease approach, whereby incidence and prevalence data are used to identify needs of the population, often through a ranking of conditions and related treatment options from most to least prevalent. This approach, taken up by the World Health Organization through the 1990s,[20] implies that more resources should go to treating those diseases which are more prevalent. Needs assessments of this form indicate the extent of different health problems but do not provide information on how much and in what manner resources should be spent.

Instead what is required is information on capacity to benefit, whereby the "return" for the resources spent, however defined, is detailed.[21,22] This is because it may be that intervening to deal with smaller problems – that is those diseases or conditions not at the top of the prevalence list – but which have particularly effective interventions available, may provide more benefits per dollar spent. An example of this is the provision of foot care for older people. In one example from the UK,[23] it was found that a podiatric intervention can provide a high level of benefit or return on investment, and that the marginal benefit is likely to exceed that of resource expenditure on other (perhaps more prevalent) conditions. It is also the case that the capacity to benefit approach specifically looks at the relevant bundle of resources and asks how that bundle can affect the problems at hand. A burden of disease approach does not normally consider this effect as it focuses on identifying the size of the problem rather than looking at the impact of the intervention relative to its costs.

A related approach which is commonly used internationally in advocating for more resources for a particular condition is that of cost of illness. In such studies, the overall cost of a particular disease is presented and compared to the overall cost of other conditions. In making such a comparison, it is implied that if one condition imposes a greater economic burden on society than its comparators, more resources should be spent on that condition. However, shifting resources based on the size of cost of illness estimates is unlikely to lead to efficient deployment of resources.[24] This is again because the size of the problem, in this case as measured by the cost, does not provide an indication of the best use of the resources available.

All this is not to say that needs assessments are not important; such data can be useful in identifying unmet need, or drawing attention to societal burdens. However, needs assessments alone are not useful for promoting the efficient use of resources, and are not best used as a primary mechanism for setting priorities. In sum, caution must be taken when reviewing a needs assessment which highlights a given service to be a priority by highlighting "need", when in fact economic arguments may indicate otherwise.

Defining core services

A third common approach to rationing in health care is for a group of decision makers or experts to attempt to define a basket of core services based on a set of criteria, and thereafter only publicly fund those services. New Zealand, the Netherlands and other countries have tried this approach for setting priorities across different treatments using criteria such as: effectiveness; efficiency; necessity; fair use of public money; and involvement of public values.[8,25,26] In practice, however, countries have had difficulty rationing services in this manner, in part due to a lack of information available for assessing how individual services meet the stated criteria. In addition, the core services approach does not necessarily lead to greater efficiency within those services which would receive public funding, as it provides no guidance on resource allocation within the "core services". In reality, the allocation within those services that are deemed to be core is likely to be based on historical patterns, which as already discussed, is off the mark in its own right.

As New Zealand represents a particularly interesting case study, a few more details of the experience with core services in this country are outlined here. In the early 1990s, the New Zealand government established a Core Services Committee which had as its aim to identify a basket of core services. Those services falling outside this basket would fall to the responsibility of individual citizens. The stated aims were to promote accountability, have a more explicit funding process, promote efficient and equitable resource allocation, provide a means to cap government expenditure, and involve the public.[25] Due to practical difficulties, however, by 1994 the focus of the Core Services Committee shifted to providing "policy guidelines" which regionalised bodies (i.e. health authorities) were to follow in setting local priorities. Thus the plan for defining a core set of services, at least at the national level, failed. It was also recognised that guidelines do not necessarily promote efficiency or equity, and that a pragmatic, economic approach for priority setting would still be required at the local and/or broader levels.[27]

From a health economics perspective, it is also important to emphasise that the core services approach ignores the notion of the margin. For example, a particular service may not be included within the core services offered, yet, for some consumers, it might provide more benefit per dollar spent than is the case for other consumers of services that are in the core. However, as those services that are not included are "out", a shifting of some resources from those services that are "in" to those that are "out" is not allowed. Overall, the core services approach as used in specific countries has had a limited effect on policy making.[6] What is needed is not a definition to support a set of core services, but rather an approach which enables decision makers to trade off service items of lower value for those of higher value. Developing a core set of services to guide funding decisions will not result in an efficient use of resources.

Accountability for Reasonableness

For any given approach to priority setting, the emphasis in the literature is on ensuring that the chosen process is fair. This can be manifested through any number of characteristics, as discussed earlier in the chapter. In order to more formally evaluate priority setting processes, an ethical framework has been developed by Daniels and Sabin called Accountability for Reasonableness.[28] The focus is not so much on the specific decisions that have to be made but rather on the process used to reach those decisions. An institution's priority setting decisions may be considered fair if they satisfy four conditions: publicity, relevance, appeals, and enforcement. These conditions, along with brief descriptions, are found in Table 3.1.

The key is in recognising that this type of ethical framework is to be applied so as to evaluate a specific approach to setting priorities. The focus here is not on the "how to", as with the three approaches to priority setting discussed earlier in the chapter, but rather is about "how fair" the process, and not necessarily the outcome, is. While initial exploration of what is involved in organisational decision making processes has been fruitful,[29] further steps are required to test more fully the usability and appropriateness of the Accountability for Reasonableness framework at different levels of healthcare decision making.

In the meantime, the four conditions would appear to provide a valuable check on any priority setting activity, in order to ensure the process or approach used is fair and transparent. Therefore, this framework can be used in conjunction with, rather than as a substitute for, almost any other approach to priority setting. As already alluded to, a

Table 3.1 Conditions of Accountability for Reasonableness framework	
Condition	**Description**
Publicity	Limit-setting decisions and their rationales must be publicly accessible
Relevance	These rationales must rest on evidence, reasons and principles that fair-minded parties (managers, clinicians, patients and consumers in general) can agree are relevant to deciding how to meet the diverse needs of a covered population under necessary resource constraints
Appeals	There is a mechanism for challenge and dispute resolution regarding limit-setting decisions, including the opportunity for revising decisions in light of further evidence or arguments
Enforcement	There is either voluntary or public regulation of the process to ensure that the first three conditions are met

further caveat is that not only should the four conditions be met, thereby ensuring the process is fair, but also that the economic concepts of opportunity cost and the margin are adhered to, so as to foster an environment through which objectives of efficiency and equity can also be achieved with the resource allocation decisions made. An example of applying the Accountability for Reasonableness framework is found in Chapter 7.

Summary

Historical allocation does not enable benefit to be maximised for the resources available. Needs assessment and related cost of illness studies, in isolation, are not sufficient for priority setting. As opportunity costs are not usually considered, and the margin is ignored, a decision mechanism for maximising benefit to the population overall is not achieved. With respect to the idea of core services, this approach also ignores the margin, and in countries where it has been applied, evidence suggests that it has had limited impact on policy making. There is no doubt that having a basket of core services is an intuitively attractive option, but for the reasons outlined, going down this path will not result in getting the most out of the resources available.

Recent contributions by researchers working with the Accountability for Reasonableness framework were also outlined in this chapter. The important distinction between this ethical framework, and the other approaches in Chapters 3 and 4, is that Accountability for Reasonableness is a framework for evaluating priority setting processes, as opposed to providing decision makers with the "nuts and bolts" to get on with priority setting. To what degree the four conditions espoused in Table 3.1 are adhered to will provide insight into how fair a given process is. Coupling this with the economic concepts of opportunity cost and the margin provides decision makers with the tools to maximise benefit, or better meet other important criteria, in a fair manner.

References

1 Breen D. Setting priorities: a framework for the assessment of health care priorities in Scottish health boards. *Health Bull* 1991;**49**:34–9.
2 Wilson H, Scott S. PBMA – its role in the future purchasing arrangements for health care services. *Health Policy* 1995;**33**:157–60.
3 Kelly K, ed. *Health Care Rationing Dilemma and Paradox*. St. Louis: Mosby, 1994.
4 Norheim O. The Norwegian welfare state in transition: rationing and plurality of values as ethical challenges for the health care system. *J Med Philos* 1995;**20**:639–55.
5 McKneally M, Dickens B, Meslin E, Singer P. Bioethics for clinicians: 13. Resource allocation. *Can Med Assoc J* 1997;**157**:163–7.
6 Maynard A, Bloor K. *Our Certain Fate: Rationing in Health Care*. London: Office of Health Economics, 1998.
7 Donaldson C, Farrar S. Needs assessment: developing an economic approach. *Health Policy* 1993;**25**:95–108.
8 Feighan T. *Setting health care priorities in Northern Ireland*. Paper presented at the Health Economists' Study Group, University of Galway, 1998.
9 Bryan S, Roberts T, Heginbotham C, McCallum A. *Public involvement in health care priority setting: an economic perspective*. Paper presented at the Health Economists' Study Group, University of Galway, 1998.
10 Robinson R. Economic evaluation and health care: the policy context. *BMJ* 1993;**307**:994–6.
11 Scott A, Donaldson C, Scott S. Program budgeting and marginal analysis: pragmatism and policy (editorial). *J Health Serv Res Policy* 1999;**4**:1–2.
12 Cohen D. Messages from Mid Glamorgan: a multi-programme experiment with marginal analysis. *Health Policy* 1995;**33**:147–55.
13 Mitton C, Donaldson C. Setting priorities in Canadian regional health authorities: a survey of key decision makers. *Health Policy* 2002;**60**:39–58.
14 Miller P. Managing informed purchasing: a survey of decision makers. *J Manage Med* 1997;**11**:35–42.

15 Vale L. *Programme Budgeting: Key Decision Makers Survey*. Aberdeen: Grampian Health Board, 1996.

16 Mooney G, Wiseman V. *Listening to the bureaucrats to establish principles for priority setting*. SPHERe Discussion Paper 1/99. Sydney: University of Sydney, 1999.

17 Birch S, Chambers S. To each according to need: a community-based approach to allocating health care resources. *Can Med Assoc J* 1993;**149**:607–12.

18 Segal L, Richardson J. *Efficiency in Resource Allocation*. Fairfield, Australia: National Centre for Health Program Evaluation, 1994.

19 Craig N, Parkin D, Gerard K. Clearing the fog on the Tyne: programme budgeting in Newcastle and North Tyneside Health Authority. *Health Policy* 1995;**33**:107–25.

20 Murray C, Lopez A. *The Global Burden of Disease*. Boston: Harvard School of Public Health, 1996.

21 Mooney G, Irwig L, Leeder S. Priority setting in health care: unburdening from the burden of disease. *Aust NZ J Public Health* 1997;**21**:680–1.

22 Culyer AJ. Equity – some theory and its policy implications. *J Med Ethics* 2001;**27**:275–83.

23 Bryan S, Parkin D, Donaldson C. Chiropody and the QALY: A case study in assigning categories of disability and distress to patients. *Health Policy* 1991;**18**:169–85.

24 Shiell A, Gerard K, Donaldson C. Cost of illness studies: an aid to decision making? *Health Policy* 1987;**8**:317–23.

25 Cumming J. Core services and priority setting: the New Zealand experience. *Health Policy* 1994;**29**:41–60.

26 Wordsworth S, Donaldson C, Scott A. *Can we afford the NHS?* London: Institute for Public Policy Research, 1996.

27 Ashton T, Cumming J, Devlin N. Priority-setting in New Zealand: translating principles into practice. *J Health Serv Res Policy* 2000;**5**:170–5.

28 Daniels N, Sabin J. The ethics of accountability in managed care reform. *Health Affairs* 1998;**17**:50–64.

29 Martin D, Pater JL, Singer P. Priority setting decisions for new cancer drugs: a qualitative case study. *Lancet* 2001;**358**:1676–81.

4: "Economic" approaches to priority setting

Introduction

Building on the approaches presented in Chapter 3, this chapter moves into a discussion of economic options for priority setting. The following approaches are presented here.

- Economic evaluation, including:
  - cost–effectiveness analysis
  - cost–benefit analysis
  - cost–utility analysis.
- Quality adjusted life year (QALY) league tables.
- Programme budgeting and marginal analysis (PBMA).

In the end, the discussion will move to recommend PBMA as the best way forward, due to its adherence to the fundamental economic concepts, its pragmatic nature in allowing decision makers to develop timely responses to pressing questions while enabling consideration of multiple inputs (such as evidence from the literature, local data and local expert opinion), and its ability to incorporate some of the other approaches outlined here, for example economic evaluation.

Economic evaluation

Economic evaluation comprises a set of techniques which enable the measurement of costs alongside benefits in assessing the potential impact of implementing ways of providing health care. Such evaluations can assist in answering questions of what to do as well as how it is best done.[1] Depending on the nature of the question involved, i.e.

whether technical or allocative efficiency is to be addressed, one of three main forms of economic evaluation can be employed.

Cost–effectiveness analysis

Cost–effectiveness analysis (CEA) is used to address questions of technical efficiency. It is applied in situations where a choice between at least two options with the same goal must be made. That is, given that a particular goal is to be achieved for a fixed budget, CEA can provide a response to the question, "What is the best way to obtain that goal?". As a result, the unit of measurement in CEA studies is generally limited to natural outcomes, or to outputs which have only one dimension, such as life years or symptom free days. While narrow in scope by definition, CEAs are frequently conducted in part because they are the simplest form of economic evaluation. A special type of CEA is cost-minimisation analysis (CMA), in which two options are deemed to have the same health outcome, leaving the analyst to solely measure differences in cost. As the assumption of equal outcomes can rarely be made, the applicability of CMA is limited.

Cost–benefit analysis

In order to address questions of allocative efficiency, that is questions of "whether" and "how much", cost–benefit analysis (CBA) can be used to assist in determining which goals are worth achieving. In other words, CBA seeks to help judgements about how much of society's resources should be allocated to a particular type of health care. In terms of opportunity cost, the question is raised as to whether the benefit to be obtained from one service is more or less than the benefit that would be obtained from alternative uses of the same resources. In order to make such comparisons, the outcome measure ideally should be measured in the same currency as costs, i.e. money. Willingness to pay is one economic technique which allows benefits to have a monetary value placed on the intervention(s) being evaluated.[2] In such studies, individuals are not being asked to make actual payments for a service, but rather their strength of preference for a particular health state or type of health care is being evaluated in monetary terms, where money is simply a measuring rod of value.

Cost–utility analysis

The third type of economic evaluation is cost–utility analysis (CUA), which can be used to examine technical or allocative efficiency. In terms of technical efficiency, CUA can inform the most efficient way to treat a particular condition, by comparing the costs per unit of health gain of different possible treatments. The option which yields the least cost per unit of health gain, or the most health gain for the same cost, is the most technically efficient. With respect to allocative efficiency, CUA can be used to make comparisons across different domains, involving some shifting of resources from one patient group to another. In order to enable such broader comparisons, the outcome measure must also be sufficiently broad. In CUA, health outcomes are measured as "healthy gains", the most common, introduced below and discussed in more detail in Chapter 10, being the QALY. This measure quantifies both quantity and quality of life in one metric. CUA is advantageous in that it uses a broad unit of benefit, and the quantification of benefit is in non-money terms. However, unlike CBA, non-health aspects of benefit, such as patient-staff interaction, waiting time and service location are beyond the scope of the CUA approach.[3]

Strengths and weaknesses

Economic evaluations have been used in many circumstances on an individual basis to inform policy decisions, and as well have been incorporated into "league tables", as discussed below. When used appropriately, the primary strengths of these evaluations are that both costs and outputs are being considered, and that two or more treatments are directly compared in terms of incremental, or marginal, gains. This ensures that change in costs and benefits are the key outcomes, thereby avoiding some of the problems of needs assessment discussed in Chapter 3.

Limitations include the significant time and cost required, rendering full blown economic evaluations not feasible for every decision that needs to be made. (Although the "way of thinking" behind the evaluations certainly is feasible in every case!) As well, these evaluations are not designed to weigh up political factors vis-à-vis efficiency, nor can they address other relevant health system objectives such as those related to equity. Finally, economic evaluations will rarely take account of all the treatment or service options a decision maker is faced with when considering questions of priority setting across a whole range of options. As such, in terms of priority setting, results from individual economic evaluations are best used as an input into a broader framework.[4]

Cost-increasing scenarios and the incremental cost–effectiveness ratio

As shown in Figure 2.2 a number of scenarios can result when assessing treatment comparators on the basis of costs and benefits. If a given treatment A results in an equal or better health outcome at less cost than treatment B, treatment A is more efficient – as in cell A1 in the matrix in Figure 2.2. If treatment A results in a better health outcome at increased cost, then some judgement is needed in weighing up whether the additional benefit is *worth* the additional cost – as in cell C1 in Figure 2.2. In the latter instance, a common output of economic evaluation studies is an incremental cost–effectiveness ratio (ICER). The ICER quantifies the incremental cost required to obtain an incremental benefit. To its detriment, study authors will often state that a given treatment is "cost-effective" because of the "favourable", or low, cost per unit of output expressed through a particular ICER.[5] In stating results in this manner, however, explicit consideration is not being given to opportunity costs.

The ICER by definition relates to extra costs required to produce the stated health gain. As the extra resources have to come from somewhere else at the expense of some other treatment or service, an opportunity cost results. Only through further examination, comparing the given treatment option with other uses of those additional resources can information be obtained about the efficiency of the treatment. In this case, the formation of an ICER moves the evaluation into the realm of allocative efficiency, and thereby ceases to be CEA despite being labelled as such.

It is also the case that despite a genuine desire for clinicians and managers to institute "cost-effective" treatments, doing so can lead to over-spending in healthcare organisations. That is, in following best practice guidelines and implementing services that are stated in the literature to be cost-effective, health organisations may unknowingly increase expenditure because resources required by those services are usually incremental to current expenditure. The message here is not about not instituting best practices, but there is a need to be cognisant that in implementing a strategy that is claimed to be cost-effective – that is one with a low ICER – expenditure will not decrease. In this context, a determination of whether a treatment is more or less cost-effective can only be made when a service which has a draw on incremental resources is compared to other potential uses of those additional resources.

As this discussion highlights, even "economic" approaches to priority setting do not always adhere to the underlying economic concept of opportunity cost at the point of application. The ICER provides an indication of how much more output results for a given amount of additional resources, but does not indicate if the extra resources required are best spent on the service or treatment under consideration. Managers, doctors and politicians the world over seem to want to buy increments of effectiveness without reference to the opportunity cost. Thus the message here is for an economic way of thinking to be encouraged, noting the potential pitfalls with ICERs. For the purposes of priority setting, individual economic evaluations are best set within a broader framework, as will be seen in Chapter 5.

Quality adjusted life year (QALY) league tables

A related approach to economic evaluation is cost per QALY league tables. With this approach, new interventions, or extensions of activity in existing interventions, are ranked in terms of their incremental cost per QALY gain.* Those items with low incremental cost per QALY gained ratios are placed, in order, at the top of the league table and those with higher ratios at the bottom. The league table is constructed through compiling results from different CUA studies, an example of which is found in Table 4.1.[6] Such a listing is based on the idea that procedures with a lower cost per QALY ratio should receive resources ahead of those with higher ratios. If additional resources are allocated to the healthcare budget, spending in accordance with the league table ranking will produce the most QALYs for those resources.

As the focus is on informing how best to spend additional resources, the margin is considered with this approach. In addition, opportunity cost is also incorporated, albeit in a constrained manner, through making explicit comparison of benefits gained and lost for the additional resources available. What the league table does not do, nor is it intended to do, is to consider how existing resources should be shifted or reallocated within the existing budget. The focus is simply on how best to spend additional resources, and within this context league tables may be a useful tool.

QALY league tables also have a number of potential limitations. As each entry in the league table is being compared with a different service or treatment, while the relative value of the item listed may be good next to its comparator, if the comparator is an inefficient treatment, the listed item will appear to be efficient even if in an absolute sense it is actually inefficient (but just not as inefficient as its comparator).[7] Further, if more benefit per pound spent could be realised by investing some or all of the additional resources in a programme not included in the league table listing, benefit overall will not be maximised. In this way, opportunity cost is considered with the league table approach, but in a more constrained way, as alternative uses of the resources outside of the league table cannot be considered.

In addition, reviews of the economic evaluation literature have found that the methods and reporting in individual studies can be inconsistent.[8] Having a ranking thus masks the limitations of the individual studies on which the league table is constructed, thereby potentially resulting in decision

---

*One QALY is best thought of as equivalent to a "healthy year".

Table 4.1 League table of costs and QALYs for selected healthcare interventions*

Intervention	Cost per QALY (1991 UK £)
Cholesterol testing and diet therapy only (all adults aged 40–69 years)	220
Neurosurgical intervention for head injury	240
General practitioner advice to stop smoking	270
Neurosurgical intervention for subarachnoid haemorrhage	490
Anti-hypertensive therapy to prevent stroke (ages 45–64 years)	940
Pacemaker implantation	1100
Valve replacement for aortic stenosis	1140
Hip replacement	1180
Cholesterol testing and treatment	1480
Coronary artery bypass graft (left main vessel disease, severe angina)	2090
Kidney transplantation	4710
Breast cancer screening	5780
Heart transplantation	7840
Cholesterol testing and treatment (incrementally) of all adults aged 25–39 years	14 150
Home dialysis	17 260
Coronary artery bypass graft (one-vessel disease, moderate angina)	18 830
Continuous ambulatory peritoneal dialysis	19 780
Hospital haemodialysis	21 970
Erythropoietin for anaemia in dialysis (assuming 10% reduction in mortality)	54 380
Neurosurgical intervention for malignant intracranial tumours	107 780
Erythropoietin for anaemia in dialysis patients (no mortality impact)	126 290

*Reproduced from Maynard (1991)[6] with permision from Blackwell publishing presented here for illustration purposes only.
QALY, quality adjusted life year.

making being based, unknowingly, on poor quality data. Another important limitation is that QALYs are limited to providing data on health benefits. If the aim is to maximise QALYs, then the league table approach can be useful, but it is more likely that broader objectives beyond QALY maximisation will be favoured. Finally, it is not clear how league tables address the issue of equity, and as such, how to allocate additional resources when a broader set of criteria beyond efficiency is to be considered.

In the end, the important point is to take caution when applying QALY league table results, recognising first that their purpose is in allocating new resources and second that a number of potential limitations can arise. What may be preferred is a more pragmatic approach which considers health and non-health benefit gain vis-à-vis costs, based on a set of criteria which includes but is not limited to efficiency, and as well enables not only additional but also current resources to be examined.

Programme budgeting and marginal analysis

Levels of application and driving questions

There is a need for a priority setting approach which allows for the complexities of healthcare decision making, and which also adheres to the economic concepts outlined in Chapter 2. One approach which meets these challenges, and which has been used widely in health care over the past 25 years, is PBMA.[9-12] The starting point of PBMA is to examine how resources are currently spent before focusing on marginal benefits and marginal costs of changes in that spend. PBMA can be used at:

- a micro level, i.e. within programmes of care
- a meso level, i.e. across services within the same general area of care
- a macro level, i.e. across all programme areas within a single health organisation.

Conceptually, the thinking could also occur at a governmental level, in planning across funded health organisations, or even inter-sectorally, across government departments like health, education and social services. At its core, the approach can be operationalised by asking five questions about resource use, as outlined in Box 4.1.

> ## Box 4.1 Five questions to operationalise PBMA
>
> 1 What are the total resources available within a given service area or health organisation?
> 2 On which services are these resources currently spent?
> 3 What services are candidates for receiving more or new resources (and what are the costs and potential benefits of putting resources into such growth areas)?
> 4 Can any existing services be provided as effectively, but with fewer resources, so releasing resources to fund items on the growth list?
> 5 If some growth areas still cannot be funded, are there any services which should receive fewer resources, or even be stopped, because greater benefit per pound spent (or a greater fit with other defined criteria) would be reached by funding the growth option as opposed to the existing service?

The first two questions relate to programme budgeting, while the last three pertain to marginal analysis. The underlying premise of programme budgeting is highlighted by the question, "How can we know where we are going if we do not know where we are?". The focus then moves to examining the effects of changes in the allocation of resources spent. That is, marginal analysis involves assessing the costs and benefits of proposed changes in the services provided and using this information to improve benefit overall. This is generally done through the formation of an advisory panel which is charged with identifying, for a given budget planning cycle, areas of service growth, and, in order to fund the proposed growth, areas for resource release. The aim is generally to make resource allocation recommendations so as to better meet a pre-defined set of criteria.

While PBMA is based on the same concepts underlying economic evaluation, it is a more pragmatic approach which enables the decision matrix described in Chapter 2 to be operationalised in a timely manner. If the budget is fixed, opportunity cost is accounted for by recognising that the items for service growth (question 3 of Box 4.1) can be funded only by taking resources from elsewhere. Resources can be obtained from elsewhere by being more technically efficient (question 4 of Box 4.1, or cells A1, A2 and B1 in Figure 2.2) or more allocatively efficient (question 5 of Box 4.1, or cells C1 and A3 in Figure 2.2). All of this can be done "at the margin" by considering the amounts of different services provided.

Of course, governments tend to add real resources incrementally to health organisation budgets year on year, and further revenue generation opportunities often exist. Many of these "new" resources will go to the top-priority growth areas (without necessarily considering how efficiency improvements could first be made within the base). Importantly, given that such increased funds are unlikely to cover all proposed growth areas, the principles of PBMA still apply. As *all* resources within or external to the given budget have an opportunity cost, the key is thus in weighing out the optimal manner to spend each resource unit used, vis-à-vis alternatives, regardless of where those units came from. As such, even when a budget is not completely fixed, the questions outlined in Box 4.1 still provide guidance in determining how best to spend available resources.

PBMA challenges

A key challenge for PBMA, and indeed other explicit approaches to priority setting, appears to be the "fit" of the approach within the context of the given organisation in which it is being applied.[13] The uptake of a formal, systematic process of setting priorities is likely to be affected by various organisational barriers and facilitators such as high level acceptance and backing, adequate resourcing, and a culture to support change. Similarly, once recommendations are made by a PBMA advisory panel, follow-through on those recommendations can also be lacking. These organisational issues are returned to in Chapter 12.

One further challenge worth mentioning at this stage, which is discussed further in Chapter 8, is that PBMA is seen as being "data hungry". While this may be the case, decisions have to be made with or without an explicit approach to priority setting. In formalising the process with PBMA, no more or less data necessarily have to be used. It is also often very difficult to estimate and value marginal benefits. Proponents of the PBMA approach would argue that it is the way of thinking provided by marginal analysis that is the key to making trade-offs explicit and improving decision making.

Thus, despite information gaps, often at times on the benefit side, this approach provides a mechanism through which priority setting and subsequent resource allocation can occur.

Summary

Economic evaluations usually consider marginal costs and benefits, and, apart from misinterpretation of ICERs, also incorporate the notion of opportunity cost. However, given the time consuming nature of such studies and their cost more generally, it is normally not possible to use economic evaluation to inform routine priority setting in health care apart from consideration of specific interventions. As such, they are likely to be more usefully encompassed within a broader priority setting framework. QALY league tables may help to divide up resources in a manner in which the most QALYs will be realised, but this is unlikely to be an objective of health organisations.

The PBMA approach provides a useful method for priority setting and has been used widely internationally. It allows for decision making to be based on the best available evidence, and in the end relies on the opinions of an advisory panel for recommending changes to the mix of services offered. As Shiell and Hall state, it is by looking at potential shifts in resources that the best balance of care can be reached.[14] By considering opportunity costs at the margin, decision makers can improve service delivery options within the constraint of limited resources. PBMA provides a means of doing this whilst taking account of the complexities of healthcare decision making.

Having critiqued a number of methods in Chapters 3 and 4 which, it could be argued, form the basis of other toolkits to be used in healthcare priority setting, in Chapter 5, a step by step guide to implementing the PBMA approach is provided. Following this, in Chapter 6, a brief history of PBMA, and further details on its application in real-world settings, is provided. In Chapter 7, specific international examples of the application of PBMA at different levels in health organisations are presented. Then, picking up on some of the issues mentioned above, in Chapters 8 through 12, a number of challenges to applying PBMA and other informed, explicit approaches to priority setting are considered, along with means of overcoming these barriers.

References

1   Auld C, Donaldson C, Mitton C, Shackley P. Economic evaluation. In: Detels R, Holland W, McEwan J, Omenn G, eds. *Oxford Textbook of Public Health, 4th edn.* Oxford: Oxford University Press, 2001.
2   Olsen JA, Donaldson C. Helicopters, hearts and hips: using willingness to pay to set priorities for public sector health care programmes. *Soc Sci Med* 1997;46:1–12.
3   Shackley P, Ryan M. Involving consumers in health care decision making. *Health Care Analysis* 1995;3:196–204.
4   Mitton C, Jarrell J. Economic evaluation in gynecology and obstetrics: principles and practice. *Can J Obstet Gynecol* 2003;25:219–23.
5   Donaldson C, Currie G, Mitton C. Contra-indications to cost effectiveness analysis in health care. *BMJ* 2002;325:891–4.
6   Maynard AK. Developing the health care market. *Econ J* 1991;101: 1277–86.
7   Birch S, Gafni A. Cost-effectiveness ratios: in a league of their own. *Health Policy* 1992;28:133–41.
8   Gerard K, Smoker I, Seymour J. Raising the quality of cost-utility analyses studies: Lessons learnt and still to learn. *Health Policy* 1999;46:217–38.
9   Twaddle S, Walker A. Programme budgeting and marginal analysis: application within programmes to assist purchasing in Greater Glasgow Health Board. *Health Policy* 1995;33:91–105.
10 Ruta D, Donaldson C, Gilray I. Economics, public health and health care purchasing: the Tayside experience of programme budgeting and marginal analysis. *J Health Serv Res Policy* 1996;1:185–93.
11 Peacock S. *An Evaluation of Program Budgeting and Marginal Analysis Applied in South Australian Hospitals.* Melbourne: Centre for Health Program Evaluation, Monash University, 1998.
12 Mitton C, Donaldson C, Halma L, Gall N. Setting priorities and allocating resources in regional health authorities: a report from two pilot exercises using program budgeting and marginal analysis *Healthcare Manage Forum* 2002;15:39.
13 Mitton C, Donaldson C. Setting priorities and allocating resources in health regions: lessons from a project evaluating program budgeting and marginal analysis (PBMA). *Health Policy* 2003;64:335–48.
14 Shiell A, Hall J. *Advancing Health in NSW: Planning in an Economic Framework.* Sydney: CHERE, 1993.

Part 3: Programme budgeting and marginal analysis (PBMA)

5: Details for implementing PBMA

Introduction

In the previous two chapters, a number of approaches to priority setting were critically appraised, specifically from a health economics perspective, through consideration of the economic concepts of opportunity cost and the margin. The conclusion from that review is that more weight must be given by decision makers to these economic concepts in priority setting activity and that one means of operationalising the concepts is through the application of PBMA. In this chapter, details are provided about the process of PBMA to enable the reader to potentially carry out an exercise on their own, or at a minimum, to know if the approach is appropriate and to get a sense of how it might best be applied in a given context.

Basic process

One of the strengths of PBMA is its adaptability to the local context, and thus it is difficult to speak of one particular way to apply the PBMA approach. That said, based on our own experience and that of others as reported in the literature, seven basic stages of PBMA can be identified and are outlined in Box 5.1. As pointed out at the end of Chapter 4, challenges, and ways of addressing these challenges, are picked up on in more detail in Chapters 8–12.

Scope and programme budget

The first step in applying PBMA is to determine the aim and scope of the priority setting activity. For example, this may be to determine optimum investment of resources across all programmes and communities in a health organisation, or alternatively to determine how best to spend resources within

Box 5.1 Stages in a PBMA priority setting exercise

1 Determine the aim and scope of the priority setting exercise
2 Compile a "programme budget", being a map of current activity and expenditure
3 Form "marginal analysis" advisory panel
4 Determine locally relevant decision making criteria

   (a) decision maker input
   (b) Board of Director input
   (c) public input

5 Advisory panel to identify options in terms of:

   (a) areas for service growth
   (b) areas for resource release through producing same level of output (or outcomes) but with less resources
   (c) areas for resource release through scaling back or stopping some services

6 Advisory panel to make recommendations in terms of:

   (a) funding growth areas with new resources
   (b) decisions to move resources from 5(b) into 5(a)
   (c) trade-off decisions to move resources from 5(c) to 5(a) if relative value in 5(c) is deemed greater than that in 5(a)

7 Validity checks with additional stakeholders and final decisions to inform budget planning process

a specific programme or service. The next step is to develop a programme budget. As discussed in more detail in Chapter 9, this is a map of the current activity and expenditure in the health organisation or given programme. In essence, the programme budget provides a starting point from which resource reallocation and service re-design options can be considered. Once the mapping is underway, an advisory panel can be formed.

Advisory panel

Careful consideration must be given to the make-up of the advisory panel. The balance is in obtaining a representative group, but also in not being overly large so as to make the decision making process unmanageable. The specific composition will be dependent on the question under consideration and the scope of the exercise. The panel may be composed of a mix of clinical personnel and managers, and could include lay membership. For application at a fairly broad level, the core advisory panel might simply be the senior management team of the health organisation. For applications within programme areas, a programme administrator and relevant clinical staff can be involved. As well, data and financial personnel are key people to have on hand, to provide support for the decision making process. Physician involvement should be encouraged in the PBMA process and is discussed in Chapter 12.

Decision making criteria

Prior to examining options for change, the panel must determine a set of decision making criteria on which the activity will be based. These criteria may reflect the values of the organisation, the health care system or society at large.* The criteria can be identified in various ways. One option would be for the decision makers to do this on their own, which may include a review of relevant business plans and other internal documents. Alternatively, input from other stakeholders, such as the Board of Directors of the given health organisation can be obtained. However, Board members are unlikely to provide good representation of the general public,[1] and in some jurisdictions such governance Boards do not exist. Thus, the public can be consulted directly, through survey work or focus groups. While democratic theory would suggest that public involvement is preferable,[2] challenges in gaining a representative sample of the population at large, and the expense of such consultations, require due consideration. These issues are discussed further in Chapter 11. Regardless of the source, it is important that the criteria be specified *a priori* and, if possible, that they are weighted to reflect the relative importance of each.

---

*Examples from the literature would include criteria such as health gain, access, innovation, sustainability, staff retention/recruitment and system integration.

Options for change

Continuing with the steps outlined in Box 5.1, once the advisory panel is set and the criteria have been identified, a prioritised list of service growth options can be developed. As well, current expenditure can be examined to determine means of improving operational efficiency. Finally, a list of options for service reduction can be developed. This process is best supported with a standardised business case template, discussed below, and can be informed through detailed review of the programme budget. In the case of setting priorities across all programmes in the given organisation, each senior manager would be required to put forth proposed areas for service growth for their programme areas, as well as to identify efficiency opportunities and options for service reduction. If the application is within a specific programme area, conceptually the steps are the same, but potential re-designs will likely be of a smaller scale and middle or frontline managers should be involved.

Importantly, options for growth and reduction should be explicitly rated against the pre-defined criteria, using available supporting evidence. For example, if health gain is a criterion, the business case should contain information on how proposed service growth items will impact health outcomes for the relevant population. Similarly, if access is a criterion, the ability for patients to receive the service must be outlined. The business case template should be designed in a manner which readily facilitates scoring against the selected criteria and be completed by the relevant managerial and clinical staff, as above, depending on the scope of the activity. While it is common for business cases in health organisations to include various details on "risks", "costs" and "benefits", to name a few, the important point here is that the business case details be lined up directly with the decision making criteria.

Scoring options

Once the rating of each option against the criteria is completed and relevant supporting information and details are inputted into the business cases, scores should then be vetted by the advisory panel. As shown in step 6(a–c) in Box 5.1, recommendations would be made by the advisory panel to first move resources from efficiency gains into growth areas, and then to examine trade-offs between items on the investment and disinvestment lists. For the latter, it is useful to construct a single combined ranking of service growth options and proposed service reduction options based on the business case assessments according to the pre-defined criteria.

For example, following rating against the decision making criteria,* service growth items A, B and C may be assessed scores of 90, 80 and 70 (out of 100), respectively, while proposed service reduction options X, Y and Z may have scores of 85, 75 and 65, respectively. Thus, the combined listing in order of preference, according to the criteria and subsequent scores, would be: A, X, B, Y, C, Z. Ranking in this manner indicates that A is the preferred option, and in order to pursue A, resources could be released from the lowest ranked service reduction option(s) currently receiving funding. As option Z is the lowest ranked item, logically, resources should first be freed from this item and put towards the highest ranked option.

If scoring in this manner is seen as too onerous a task, a simpler application of the same concepts would be to take each service growth option and make comparisons one by one against options proposed for service reduction. In this case this would mean starting with option A and making an explicit assessment of relative value against X, Y and Z. Thus, assuming costs of expansions and reductions are equal, the group might compare A with Z and decide to reallocate from the latter to the former. This process of comparing items on the expansion list with those on the reduction list should continue until it is decided that no more gain would be had by switching resources between options. Multi-criteria decision analysis software can be used within the decision making framework once criteria have been selected and weighted.[3] Using such software does not alleviate the need for decisions to be made, but can help to organise the investment and disinvestment options and facilitate the decision making process.

---

*Rating can be done with qualitative terms such as high, medium and low, or more quantitatively on a scale from 0 to 10 or 0 to 100. Weighting is done *a priori*, and each criterion weight would be multiplied by the score given to the option under consideration. For example, if two criteria – health gain and access – were being used, option A might score 85/100 on health gain and 95/100 on access. If the criteria were weighted equally (i.e. each given a weight of 0.5), option A would receive a total score of 90 out of 100. As can be imagined, vetting of the scores by the advisory panel becomes critical.

The notion of freeing resources through improving operational efficiency is common place in health organisations. The much more challenging task, addressed further in Chapter 9, is to obtain resource releases through actual service reductions and disinvestments. As stated above, however, the logic is clear: if service growth options cannot be wholly funded through new monies and revenue generation, and operational efficiency gains have been exhausted, then some services must be scaled back or stopped in order for additional growth items to be pursued. It is also the case that proposed service reduction items are not necessarily "bad" in their own right, and indeed may be producing some value (for example option X above, having received a score of 85/100, obviously has merit). The point here, just as was made with the examples at the end of Chapter 2, is that if a service reduction option is producing less value than a service growth option *at the margin*, resources should be shifted accordingly.

Supporting evidence and information

In order to support the PBMA process, information can be obtained from available sources (Figure 5.1),[4] including evidence from the literature, local research projects, regional or state policies and guidelines, local utilisation data, informal input from staff, clinicians and members of the public, and reports from the ministry, to name just a few. In order to derive information on benefit, available evidence can be drawn upon from the literature, or patients and members of the public can be directly consulted using techniques such as those described in Chapters 10 and 11. As already stated, this supporting information should be put into the standardised business cases; if information is obtained on a particular service option that does not inform the rating assessment of one of the decision making criteria, either the information should be omitted or the criteria need to be re-thought. Guidelines can be drawn up within the organisation providing details on the various sources of information available, and how this information is best used. Explicitly laying out the compiled evidence in a business case format, with specific reference to the criteria, will foster comparative assessment of options as outlined above.

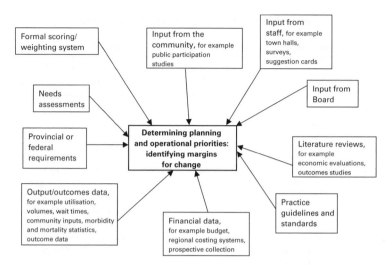

Figure 5.1 Data inputs for the priority setting process. Reprinted from Mitton C *et al*. Priority setting in health authorities: a novel approach to a historical activity. *Soc Sci Med* 2003;**57**:1655, with permission from Elsevier.

No matter how much or how little actual evidence is available, in the end the members of the advisory panel are responsible for making recommendations as to whether resources should be shifted.)[5] As will be discussed in Chapter 8, where evidence is lacking, group members can base recommendations on their own "expert" opinion. Importantly, many decisions are currently made (often implicitly) in lieu of formal evidence. The PBMA approach, as described herein, makes the process transparent, enables explicit comparison of options based on set criteria, and provides a forum through which various pieces of information can be considered by the relevant decision makers. As a final check (see Box 5.1), the last stage of PBMA is to conduct a round of consultations with a wider group of relevant stakeholders, including clinicians or members of the public not directly involved in the process, in order to test the validity of the recommendations. At this point, any concerns can be taken back to the advisory panel and final decisions made.

Table 5.1 Specific points to consider for PBMA exercises

Point to consider	Ideal time to address	Rationale
Strategically select the first PBMA exercise in a health organisation in an area where there is a confirmed champion and an "easy-win"	Prior to specific applications being selected	Need champion for group buy-in and follow-through of recommendations; early success will aid in the organisational uptake of the approach
Advisory panel should have representation from key stakeholders but not too large to prevent decision making (7–10 for micro activity and up to 20 max. for macro activity)	At the outset of the given exercise	Need to be able to get group consensus for decisions, but do not want to exclude important players; group dynamics in the process becomes critical
Use the introductory session to communicate underlying economic concepts and specifically what the application plan is	At the outset of the given exercise	Panel members have to understand opportunity cost for buy-in; provides opportunity to adjust the plan early on
Advisory panel meetings held at 2–4-week intervals	Throughout the PBMA process	Need adequate time to review literature and do background work but do not want a drawn out process; complete in <6 months
Develop a base-criteria listing (or set of principles) on which priority decisions will be made and bring this to the group for consideration	Prior to second meeting, for discussion at the second meeting	There are a limited number of criteria used in this type of decision making found in the literature; saves time by starting with a base
Consider using one-on-one meetings with panel members and ensure that each member knows that	Throughout the PBMA process	Each panel member thinks differently, needs different amounts of information, and not

(Continued)

Table 5.1 (Continued)

Point to consider	Ideal time to address	Rationale
the facilitators are open for discussion at any time		all may feel comfortable presenting a view in the large group
Put less emphasis on having all the "data" to support a decision and more on drawing out opinions from the expert group	Particularly in the later sessions of the process	Data can only take the group so far and can be used as a crutch not to make a decision; ultimately group needs to have confidence in making their own recommendations
Earmark resources (i.e. staff time) to enact the panel recommendations	Stated at the outset, carried out following the exercise	Recommendations by themselves will not see action without dedicated resources to move them forward

Lessons for applying PBMA

Through the application of PBMA in three health authorities in Alberta, Canada, a number of specific lessons for the application of the process have been compiled.[6] Considering these lessons (shown in Table 5.1) will aid in facilitating a positive impact on decision making processes. Some of these points were raised by researchers in observing the PBMA case studies, and others came directly from the users of the approach, through follow up survey work with managers and clinicians.

Summary

In focusing on resource *re*allocation, improvements to current expenditure can be realised over time. PBMA provides an explicit mechanism for operationalising the economic principles of opportunity cost and the margin. Further, this approach helps to ensure a transparent priority setting process, allows for broad consultation of allocation recommendations, enables public input to be incorporated and is driven jointly by local opinion and available evidence. The Toolkit now turns to provide a detailed history of the use of PBMA internationally, and, picking up on issues raised here, to begin to provide more detailed guidance on how this type of approach can be set within the organisational context in which it is being applied.

References

1 Frankish J, Dwan B, Ratner P, Wharf Higgins J, Larsen C. Challenges of citizen participation in regional health authorities. *Soc Sci Med* 2002;**54**:1471–80.
2 Litva A, Coast J, Donovan J *et al.* "The public is too subjective": public involvement at different levels of health-care decision making. *Soc Sci Med* 2002;**54**:1825–37.
3 Mabin V, King G, Menzies M, Joyce K. Public sector priority setting using decision support tools. *Aust J Public Administration* 2001;**60**:44–59.
4 Mitton C, Patten S, Waldner H, Donaldson C. Priority setting in health authorities: a novel approach to a historical activity. *Soc Sci Med* 2003; **57**:1653–63.
5 Peacock S. *An Evaluation of Program Budgeting and Marginal Analysis Applied in South Australian Hospitals*. Melbourne: Centre for Health Program Evaluation, Monash University, 1998.
6 Mitton C, Donaldson C. Setting priorities and allocating resources in health regions: lessons from a project evaluating program budgeting and marginal analysis (PBMA). *Health Policy* 2003;**64**:335–48.

6: Evolution of PBMA and organisational processes

Introduction

This chapter builds on the description of programme budgeting and marginal analysis (PBMA) presented in Chapters 4 and 5, by first providing a brief history and details of its use to date. This includes a full listing of publications and known unpublished papers on PBMA, classified in terms of areas of application, date and location. Following this, information is provided on what is known of the impact of real-life PBMA applications. Finally, factors for successful implementation of the approach are presented. Through this, a number of organisational barriers and facilitators of an explicit, evidence-based approach to priority setting are put forth.

Brief history of PBMA

In terms of government-funded activity, programme budgeting was first developed for use in the US defence sector in the 1950s and 1960s, as a means of tabulating expenditure data in different forms to provide information on what was being spent and in what manner. In the mid-1970s, Pole[1] recognised the applicability of programme budgeting for use in the health sector and attempted to apply the tool in Britain's Department of Health and Social Security. As programme budgeting was never meant as a tool for programme appraisal, other techniques such as cost-effectiveness analysis (CEA) and cost-benefit analysis (CBA) were recommended for use in Britain, alongside of the information framework, so that options for change could be evaluated.[2] Later, "marginal analysis" came to be understood as a broadly defined evaluative technique which could incorporate such specific types of analyses as CEA and CBA.

As a whole, however, in the 1970s, there was resistance to formal planning approaches in health care, in part because managers were unwilling to accept that resources were scarce and needs were not finite. Further, with the existence of many different levels of decision making and many different decision makers, the layered structure of the British National Health Service (NHS) was not conducive to one framework permeating all levels for use in a widespread and systematic manner. As a result, even with the introduction of explicit approaches like PBMA in the 1970s and early 1980s, priority setting decisions for the most part continued to be made on an ad hoc basis, with planning often being a response to past decisions and choices.[2]

In the early 1990s, Mooney et al.[3] stated that PBMA was becoming increasingly important, apparently aided by the introduction of the purchaser–provider split in the NHS in 1991. The attribution to this split may be too direct, however. It has been argued, for example, that the resurgence of PBMA was in part due to the clearer definition of roles between health authorities and providers,[4] and that explicit priority setting was less easily avoided by health authorities.[5] Furthermore, some of the demand would have been stimulated by managers searching around for tools and approaches to aid them in their new roles, and by health economists vying to practise their trade!

The view that a purchaser–provider split is not necessary for PBMA to have relevance to decision makers is also supported by others. What is required is an environment, as found with most health organisations, where questions are raised regarding how best to prioritise services and allocate limited resources.[6] This view is supported with the recent expansion of PBMA applications in regionalised contexts internationally where no formal internal markets exist. Further, by the early 1990s, a cultural shift was under way from implicit to explicit rationing, and with it the proliferation of economic techniques and approaches to priority setting. These developments, coupled with a more widely recognised understanding that the claims on resources vastly outstrip resource availability, have led to increased attention to and use of PBMA in recent years.[7]

For example, the application of PBMA in Australia and New Zealand has increased radically since the early 1990s. While it may be that such activity is directly related to the presence of health economists actively pursuing priority setting and

PBMA research, it would also seem that one-off exercises build on each other, as institutional knowledge of the PBMA approach grows. Based on work conducted in the UK, the journal *Health Policy* devoted an entire issue in 1995 to the use of PBMA. This in turn spawned further important "milestone" papers such as Ruta *et al.*,[8] which began to present PBMA more as a pragmatic management tool that draws in multifaceted information to support the decision making process.

The work by Ruta *et al.*[8] in Tayside, Scotland, discussed in more detail in Chapter 7, also started to develop the notion of public input into priority setting activity through the PBMA approach. This served as a parallel to other health services research examining this same issue.[9] By 1998, published accounts of PBMA activity in eastern Australia appeared,[10] and it was here that the importance of identifying a set of prerequisites or factors for success of a PBMA exercise surfaced. These efforts were picked up in Alberta, Canada, first through the application and evaluation of a series of one-off micro PBMA exercises, then with the institution of a macro level PBMA exercise at the level of a single health authority across major service areas, as described in Chapter 7.

Throughout this history, numerous challenges have arisen to the application and longer term "success" of PBMA, such as the approach being time and data intensive, how resource releases can be identified, and the "fit" of the approach within the organisational context in which it is being applied. These challenges serve as the basis for the material presented in Chapters 8 through 12, although it should be noted that these are not always specific to PBMA *per se*. It is suggested that any explicit, evidence-based approach that is based on the concepts of opportunity cost and the margin will in some way be challenged by the issues raised. Thus the discussions in these later chapters of the Toolkit extend beyond the PBMA approach.

Use of PBMA internationally

Noting this history of PBMA, it is also useful for decision makers and academics alike to have a sense of where, specifically, the approach has been applied, as well as the impact of the approach including whether its use was sustained beyond the specific applications reported.

Application of PBMA

A recent study sought to categorise previous PBMA exercises, and determine the short and longer term impact of PBMA in health organisations internationally.[7] Through searches in peer-review and grey literature databases, as well as through a semi-structured mail-out survey of 30 authors of PBMA studies, the use of PBMA up until 1999 was determined. A similar set of searches was then conducted to update this review to March 2003. In total, 109 published papers on PBMA were identified (see Appendix A), with the approach having been used almost 90 times in over 70 health organisations or other related contexts, in seven countries. About 10% of the exercises occurred during or before 1991, about 80% between 1992 and 2003, and the specific dates for about 10% of the exercises were unknown. Details of the exercises, including the date and type of activity, are found in Appendix B.

Impact of PBMA

The survey referred to above also provided insight into the impact of the approach on priority setting decisions. Of those where this was known, use of PBMA was reported to have continued beyond the initial reported exercise in about half the health organisations. Some of the reasons provided for the approach being discontinued included:

- change in health organisation personnel or agendas from time when it was used
- no champion to continue the PBMA cause
- health economist no longer working with the health organisation
- personnel time or money no longer earmarked for PBMA.

Overall, across the different countries, of those for which respondents of the survey knew the outcome, about 60% were reported to have had a positive short or long term impact, in that either priorities were set or resources were realigned due to using the PBMA approach. Unfortunately, it was not possible with this survey to determine the impact of PBMA on changes in the way of thinking in the regions. That is, even if

PBMA *per se* was no longer being used, it is not known if the concepts behind the approach – that is thinking about opportunity cost at the margin – were incorporated. The impact of PBMA does not appear to hinge on the availability of relevant utilisation or costing data.

Organisational issues

As already alluded to, successful implementation of PBMA relies in part on continuity of personnel and the involvement of a PBMA "champion". Further, in order for PBMA to be integrated into the culture of the organisation, the given priority setting exercise should be at least broadly consistent with ongoing activities carried out by decision makers. To expect managers and clinicians, working in an often reactive and stressful environment, to adjust their practices to incorporate an external framework is not realistic. Not only is it helpful to point out that PBMA-like activity may already be underway, thus not requiring the paradigm shift managers may initially think is required, it is also critical to build on the flexibility of PBMA and cater to specific managerial needs. A clear and quick PBMA application, with valid and useful information disseminated widely within the health organisation may serve as a valuable starting point.

Further to the key lessons learned from the body of work conducted in Alberta, Canada, as depicted in Table 5.1, a model of the PBMA process was constructed based on this work,[11] and is depicted in gradually more complex forms in Figures 6.1–6.3. These draw out some of the empirically observed organisational barriers and facilitators to the uptake of the approach and ultimate follow-through of recommendations, and also highlight issues for the development and application of PBMA as a practical decision making aid. The placement of the specific factors in the model arose from observation of the seven case studies in Alberta.

The initial model, shown in Figure 6.1, is meant to portray a number of "inputs" which should be in place for the PBMA process to be conducted. Without any one of these, application of the approach may still proceed, but success is more likely if all are present for a given application. Under the "PBMA process" box are a number of the key lessons learned (see Table 5.1).

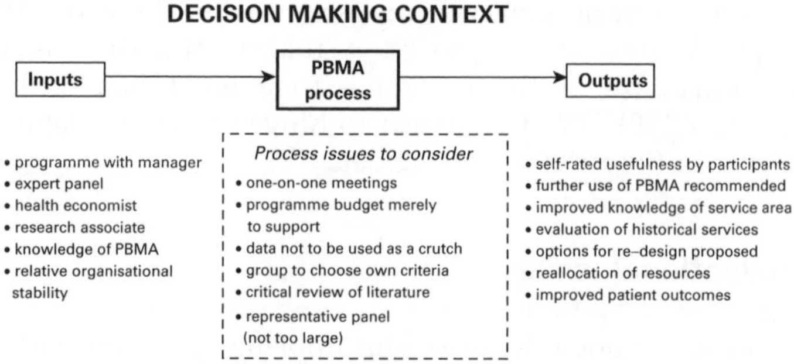

DECISION MAKING CONTEXT

Figure 6.1 Input-output model for PBMA

These illustrate that sound methodology must be applied for the process to move forward. From there, numerous potential "outputs" result from any given PBMA process. As would be expected this includes resource reallocation and improved patient outcomes, but also includes further items such as the evaluation of historical services and improved knowledge of a given service area. The outputs were generated from decision makers who have used PBMA, and begin to move the understanding of PBMA from a purely economic technique concerned with measuring marginal costs and benefits, to a management process still based on economic concepts but which contributes to strategic planning.

Barriers and facilitators to the PBMA process were also empirically observed and are included in the model. As depicted in Figure 6.2, barriers and facilitators can arise early on in the process. These factors relate to the uptake by an organisation or specific programme of an explicit approach to priority setting. In addition, as highlighted in Figure 6.3, barriers and facilitators can also arise closer to completion, and are inserted in the model following the actual PBMA process box, but prior to the outputs being achieved. These factors suggest that even if a PBMA process is conducted in an appropriate manner, there is still the likelihood that the desired outputs may not be realised. Obviously this is largely dependent on the management of the barriers and facilitators.

The depiction of barriers and facilitators in this manner actually has its roots in psychology, whereby Lewin examined factors influencing change in individuals, and coined the term "force field analysis".[12] These organisational issues are

DECISION MAKING CONTEXT

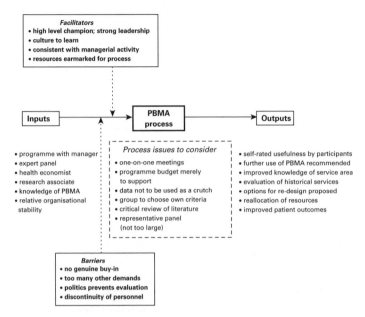

Figure 6.2 Input-output model for PBMA with barriers and facilitators depicted prior to the actual process

revisited in Chapter 12, where observations from other PBMA activity are compared to the model presented here and ties are drawn to the broader healthcare management literature. The key point to take from the model as a whole is that while a PBMA exercise can be conducted perfectly in a "technical" sense, an understanding of the context is required for the exercise to have a chance at being successful.

Summary

PBMA has been used widely internationally and provides a process to guide decision makers in making choices amongst competing claims on limited resources. In applying such an approach, organisational and managerial barriers are likely to arise. Due consideration should be given to addressing potential barriers before embarking on the process of resource

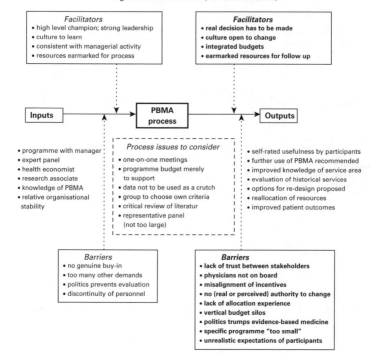

DECISION MAKING CONTEXT
Integrated delivery system (regionalisation)
Organisational behaviour (barriers/facilitators)

Figure 6.3 Input-output model for PBMA with barriers and facilitators depicted prior to and following the actual process. Reprinted with permission from Mitton and Donaldson (2003), p. 342.[11]

allocation. What is now required is to take these more theoretical discussions and provide illustrations of PBMA in practice. This is the purpose of Chapter 7, in which examples are given of the use of PBMA at two different levels in health organisations in Britain and Canada.

References

1 Pole D. Programs, priorities and budgets. *Br J Prev Soc Med* 1974;**28**:191–5.
2 Gray A, Steele R. Programme budgeting in the health sector. *Int J Manage Sci* 1979;7:451–8.

3   Mooney G, Gerard K, Donaldson C, Farrar S. *Priority setting in purchasing: some practical guidelines*. Research paper number 6. London: National Association of Health Authorities and Trusts, 1992.

4   Ratcliffe J, Donaldson C, Macphee S. Programme budgeting and marginal analysis: a case study of maternity services. *J Public Health Med* 1996;**18**:175–82.

5   Donaldson C. Economics, public health and health care purchasing: reinventing the wheel? *Health Policy* 1995;**33**:79–90.

6   Madden L, Hussey R, Mooney G, Church E. Public health and economics in tandem: programme budgeting, marginal analysis and priority setting in practice. *Health Policy* 1995;**33**:161–8.

7   Mitton C, Donaldson C. Twenty-five years of programme budgeting and marginal analysis in the health sector, 1974–1999. *J Health Serv Res Policy* 2001;**6**:239–48.

8   Ruta D, Donaldson C, Gilray I. Economics, public health and health care purchasing: the Tayside experience of programme budgeting and marginal analysis. *J Health Serv Res Policy* 1996;**1**:185–93.

9   Lomas J, Abelson J. In search of informed input: a systematic approach to involving the public in community decision making. *Healthcare Manage Forum* 1996;**9**:48–52.

10 Peacock S. *An Evaluation of Program Budgeting and Marginal Analysis Applied in South Australian Hospitals*. Melbourne: Center for Health Program Evaluation, Monash University, 1998.

11 Mitton C, Donaldson C. Setting priorities and allocating resources in health regions: lessons from a project evaluating program budgeting and marginal analysis (PBMA). *Health Policy* 2003;**64**:335–48.

12 Lewin K. *Field Theory in Social Science: Selected Theoretical Papers*. New York: Harper, 1951.

Appendix A: Publications on PBMA until March 2003

1 Alexander K, Bruggermann K. Program budgeting and marginal analysis: lessons learned from the practical application of PBMA at the Women's and Children's Hospital, South Australia, 1998.

2 Ashton T, Cumming J, Devlin N. Priority-setting in New Zealand: translating principles into practice. *J Health Serv Res Policy* 2000;**5**:170–5.

3 Astley J, Wake-Dyster W. Evidence-based priority setting. *Aust Health Rev* 2001;**24**:32–9.

4 Bohmer P, Pain C, Watt A, Abernethy P, Sceats J. Maximising health gain within available resources in the New Zealand public health system. *Health Policy* 2001;**55**:37–50.

5 Boyne D, Steele R. *Laboratory costs and programme budgeting.* Discussion paper 05/80. Aberdeen: Health Economics Research Unit, University of Aberdeen, 1980.

6 Brambleby P. *A framework for programme budgeting and commissioning at locality level in East Sussex.* Presented at the joint meeting of the Faculty of Public Health Medicine and the Health Economists' Study Group. York: University of York, 1993.

7 Brambleby P. A survivor's guide to programme budgeting. *Health Policy* 1995;**33**:127–45.

8 Breen D. Setting priorities: a framework for the assessment of health care priorities in Scottish health boards. *Health Bull* 1991;**49**:34–9.

9 Breen D. *Priority Setting Framework 1999/2000.* Dumfries and Galloway: Dumfries and Galloway Health Board, Department of Public Health Medicine, 1999.

10 Buchan S, Mooney G. *Pharmacy costs and programme budgeting.* Discussion paper 04/80. Aberdeen: Health Economics Research Unit, University of Aberdeen, 1980.

11 Carter R, Stone C, Vos T *et al. Trial of Program Budgeting and Marginal Anaylsis (PBMA) to assist cancer control planning in Australia.* Victoria, Australia: Centre for Health Program Evaluation, 2000.

12 Cohen D. Marginal analysis in practice: an alternative to needs assessment for contracting health care. *BMJ* 1994;**309**:781–5.

13 Cohen D. Messages from Mid Glamorgan: a multi-programme experiment with marginal analysis. *Health Policy* 1995;**33**:147–55.

14 Cohen D, Davies P. Priority setting in Mid Glamorgan: applying marginal analysis. *Br J Healthcare Manage* 1995;**1**:455–7.

15 Craig N, Mordue A, Parkin D, Gough H, McCann K. Tools for making purchasing decisions in district health authorities: the return of programme budgeting and marginal analysis. *Manage Economia Sanitaria* 1993;**2**:19–30.

16 Craig N, Parkin D, Gerard K. Clearing the fog on the Tyne: programme budgeting in Newcastle and North Tyneside Health Authority. *Health Policy* 1995;**33**:107–25.

17 Crockett A, Cranston J, Scown P, Moss J. *Respiratory unit program based marginal analysis: prevention and care of chronic airflow limitation,* Final report. Australia: Flinders Medical Centre Respiratory Unit, 1998.

18 Crockett A, Cranston J, Moss J, Scown P, Mooney G, Alpers J. Program budgeting and marginal analysis: a case study in chronic airflow limitation. *Aust Health Rev* 1999;**22**:65–77.

19 Davis P. *Programme Budgeting and Marginal Analysis: the Experience of West Pennine Health Authority.* York: University of York, 1994.

20 Davis P, Street A, Posnett J. *Program budgeting: a disease based approach to describing health care activity and expenditure.* Report P2002b. York: York Health Economics Consortium, University of York, 1995.

21 Donaldson C. Commentary: possible road to efficiency in the health service. *BMJ* 1994;**309**:784–5.

22 Donaldson C. Economics, public health and health care purchasing: reinventing the wheel? *Health Policy* 1995;**33**:79–90.

23 Donaldson C, Mooney G. Needs assessment, priority setting, and contracts for health care: an economic view. *BMJ* 1991;**303**:1529–30.

24 Donaldson C, Farrar S. Needs assessment: developing an economic approach. *Health Policy* 1993;**25**:95–108.

25 Donaldson C, Walker A, Craig N. *Programme Budgeting and Marginal Analysis: A Handbook for Applying Economics in Health Care Purchasing.* Glasgow: Scottish Forum for Public Health Medicine, 1995.

26 Donaldson C, Mitton C, Martin H *et al. Priority Setting within Regional Funding Envelopes: The Use of Program Budgeting and Marginal Analysis.* Ottawa: Canadian Health Services Research Foundation, 2001.

27 Donaldson C, Currie G, Mitton C. *Managing Medicare: The Prerequisite to Spending or Reform.* Toronto: CD Howe Institute, 2002.

28 Edwards D, Peacock S, Carter R. *Setting Priorities in South Australian Community health III: Regional Applications of Program Budgeting and Marginal Analysis.* Melbourne: Centre for Health Program Evaluation, Monash University, 1998.

29 Edwards D, Peacock S, Carter R. Beyond the individual: benefits and community health. In: Baldry J, ed. *Australian Health Economics Society.* Proceedings of the 20th Annual Australian Conference of Health Economists, Sydney, 1998.

30 Epidemiology Unit South West Centre for Public Health. *Asthma services across south west New South Wales: program budgeting and marginal analysis.* NSW: South West Centre for Public health, Greater Murray Health Service, 1997.

31 Firth C. Base year expenditure analysis for program budgeting in a regional health authority. *Hosp Health Serv Rev* 1979;**75**:12–18.

32 Fordyce J, Mooney G, Russel E. Economic analysis in health care: 1. The tools of evaluation; 2. An application to care of the elderly. *Health Bull* 1981;**39**:21–38.

33 Fuller J, Bentley M, Shotton D. Use of community health needs assessment for regional planning in country South Australia. *Aust J Rural Health* 2001;**9**:12–17.

34 Gold L, Raftery J, Soderlund N. *Costing diseases at DHA level: a standardised approach?* Presented at Health Economists' Study Group. York, 1997.

35 Gray A, Steele R. Programme budgeting in the health sector. *Int J Manage Sci* 1979;**7**:451–8.

36 Haas M, Mooney G, Viney R, Cooper L. Program budgeting and marginal analysis in NSW. *NSW Public Health Bull* 1997;**8**:81–3.

37 Haas M, Viney R, Kristensen E, Pain C, Foulds K. Using programme budgeting and marginal analysis to assist population based strategic planning for coronary heart disease. *Health Policy* 2001;**55**:173–86.

38 Halma L, Mitton C, Donaldson C, West B. A case study on priority setting in rural southern Alberta: keeping the house from blowing in. *Can J Rural Med* 2003 (in press).

39 Henderson LR, Scott A. The costs of caring for stroke patients in a GP-led community hospital: an application of programme budgeting and marginal analysis. *Health Soc Care Community* 2001;**9**:244–54.

40 Issaka-Tinorgah A, Waddington C. Encouraging efficiency through programme and functional budgeting: lessons from experience in Ghana and Gambia. In: Mills A, Lee K, eds. *Health economics research in developing countries.* Oxford: Oxford University Press, 1993.

41 Jan S. Institutional considerations in priority setting: transactions cost perspective on PBMA. *Health Economics* 2000;**9**:631–41.

42 Jones C, Wright K. *Programme Budgeting Revisited: Special Reference to People with Learning Disabilities.* York: York Centre for Health Economics, University of York, 1995.

43 Leeder S, Shiell A. Marginal reallocation in pursuit of more efficient health care. *Med J Aust* 1994;**160**:472–5.

44 Lees A. Improving services in a Glasgow maternity hospital. *Br J Midwifery* 1996;**4**:191–203.

45 Liverpool Health Authority. *Programme Budgeting and Marginal Analysis for Coronary Heart Disease*. Liverpool: Liverpool Health Authority, 1997.

46 Liverpool Health Authority. *Setting Priorities for Stroke*. Liverpool: Liverpool Health Authority, 1997.

47 Liverpool Health Authority. *Respiratory Disease Project*. Liverpool: Liverpool Health Authority, 1998.

48 Liverpool Health Authority. *Respiratory Project: Report on Management of Asthma in Children*. Liverpool: Liverpool Health Authority, 1998.

49 Lockett T, Raftery J, Richards J. *The strengths and limitations of programme budgeting: a district's experience*, presented at Health Economists' Study Group. Bristol University, 1995.

50 Madden L, Hussey R, Mooney G, Church E. Public health and economics in tandem: programme budgeting, marginal analysis and priority setting in practice. *Health Policy* 1995;**33**:161–68.

51 McCarthy M. The contracting round: achieving health gain or financial balance. *J Public Health Med* 1998;**20**:409–13.

52 Miller P. Managing informed purchasing: a survey of decision makers. *J Manage Med* 1997;**11**:35–42.

53 Miller P, Vale L. Programme approach to managing informed commissioning. *Health Serv Manage Res* 2001;**14**:159–64.

54 Miller P, Parkin D, Lewis D, Gerard K. Final report of the project *Developing Programme Budgeting and Marginal Analysis in Purchasing Organisations*. Newcastle: University of Newcastle upon Tyne, 1995.

55 Miller P, Parkin D, Craig N, Lewis D, Gerard K. Less fog on the Tyne? Programme budgeting in Newcastle and North Tyneside. *Health Policy* 1997;**40**:217–29.

56 Miller P, Scott A, Craig N, Walker A, Hanlon P. *Understanding the Shifts between Primary and Secondary Care in Scotland and Implications for Future Policy*. Glasgow: Scottish Forum for Public Health Medicine, 1997.

57 Miller P, Craig N, Scott A, Walker A, Hanlon P. Measuring progress towards a primary care-led NHS. *Br J Gen Pract* 1999;**49**:541–5.

58 Mitton C, Donaldson C. Twenty-five years of programme budgeting and marginal analysis in the health sector, 1974–1999. *J Health Serv Res Policy* 2001;**6**:239–48.

59 Mitton C, Donaldson C. Setting priorities in Canadian regional health authorities: A survey of key decision makers. *Health Policy* 2002;**60**:39–58.

60 Mitton C, Donaldson C. Setting priorities and allocating resources in health regions: lessons from a project evaluating program budgeting and marginal analysis (PBMA). *Health Policy* 2003;**64**:335–48.

61 Mitton C, Donaldson C, Dean S, West B. Program budgeting and marginal analysis: a priority-setting framework for Canadian Regional Health Authorities. *Healthcare Manage Forum* 2000;**13**:24–31.

62 Mitton C, Donaldson C, Halma L, Gall N. Setting priorities and allocating resources in regional health authorities: a report from two pilot exercises using program budgeting and marginal analysis. *Healthcare Manage Forum* 2002;**15**:39.

63 Mitton C, McGregor J, Conroy M, Waddell C. Making choices in health care: the reality of scarcity. *Hosp Q* 2002;**6**:48–54.

64 Mitton C, Donaldson C, Shellian B, Pagenkopf C. Priority setting in a Canadian surgical department: a case study using program budgeting and marginal analysis. *Can J Surg* 2003;**46**:23–9.

65 Mitton C, Donaldson C, Waldner H, Eagle C. The evolution of PBMA: towards a macro-level priority setting framework for health regions. *Health Care Manage Sci* 2003;**16**:96–105.

66   Mitton C, Donaldson C, Manderville P. Priority setting in a Canadian long-term care setting: a case study using program budgeting and marginal analysis. *Can J Aging* 2003 (in press).

67   Mitton C, Patten S, Waldner H, Donaldson C. Priority setting in health authorities: a novel approach to a historical activity. *Soc Sci Med* 2003; **57**:1653–63.

68   Mooney G. Programme budgeting in an area health board. *Hosp Health Serv Rev* 1977;**November:**379–84.

69   Mooney G. Planning for balance of care of the elderly. *Scottish J Political Economics* 1978;**25**:149–64.

70   Mooney G. Program budgeting: an aid to planning and priority setting in health care. *Effective Health Care* 1984;**2**:65–8.

71   Mooney G, Newberry G. Priority setting in dentistry: putting teeth into the process. *NSW Public Health Bull* 1999;**10**:42–3.

72   Mooney G, Russell E, Weir R. *Choices for Health Care: A Practical Introduction to the Economics of Health Provision.* London: Macmillan, 1986.

73   Mooney G, Gerard K, Donaldson C, Farrar S. *Priority Setting in Purchasing: some Practical Guidelines.* Research paper number 6. London: National Association of Health Authorities and Trusts, 1992.

74   Mooney G, Madden L, Hussey R. *Priority Setting in Purchasing: Public Health and Economics in Tandem,* presented at Health Economists' Study Group. York, 1993.

75   Mooney G, Jan S, Seymour J. The NSW health outcomes initiative and economic analysis. *Aust J Public Health* 1994;**18**:244–8.

76   Mooney G, Haas M, Viney R, Cooper L. *Linking Health Outcomes to Priority Setting, Planning and Resource Allocation.* NSW, Australia: Center for Health Economics Research and Evaluation, 1997.

77   Newberry G. *Setting Health Priorities: The Use of Programme Budgeting and Marginal Analysis by the Central Coast AHS.* NSW, Australia: Central Coast Area Health Service, 1996.

78   North Western Adelaide Health Service. *Implementation of program budgeting and marginal analysis 1996/97.* Final report. Adelaide: Strategic Planning and Development, NWAHS, 1998.

79   NSW Health Department. *Asthma Services Across SW NSW: Program Budgeting and Marginal Analysis.* Sydney: NSW Health Department, 1997.

80   Peacock S. *An Evaluation of Program Budgeting and Marginal Analysis Applied in South Australian Hospitals.* Melbourne: Centre for Health Program Evaluation, Monash University, 1998.

81   Peacock S. *Program Budgeting and Marginal Analysis. Options for Health Sector Reform.* Melbourne: Centre for Health Program Evaluation, Monash University, 1998.

82   Peacock S, Edwards D. *Setting Priorities in South Australian Community Health: The Mental Health Program Budget.* Melbourne: Centre for Health Program Evaluation, Monash University, 1997.

83   Peacock S, Richardson J. *PBMA in South Australia: Setting priorities in community health.* Presented at Health Economists' Study Group. Sheffield, 1998.

84   Peacock S, Richardson J, Carter R. *Setting Priorities in South Australian Community Health II: Marginal Analysis of Mental Health Service.* Melbourne: Centre for Health Program Evaluation, Monash University, 1997.

85   Plant P, Davies G, Brambleby P, Turner D. *A Standardised Approach to Programme Budgeting.* Tunbridge Wells: South East Institute of Public Health, 1995.

86   Pole J. Programs, priorities and budgets. *Br J Prev Soc Med* 1974;**28**:191–5.

87   Posnett J, Street A. Programme budgeting and marginal analysis: an approach to priority setting in need of refinement. *J Health Serv Res Policy* 1996;**1**:147–53.

88 Ratcliffe J, Donaldson C, Macphee S. Programme budgeting and marginal analysis: a case study of maternity services. *J Public Health Med* 1996;**18**:175–82.

89 Robinson R. Economic evaluation and health care: the policy context. *BMJ* 1993;**307**:994–6.

90 Ruta D, Donaldson C, Gilray I. Economics, public health and health care purchasing: the Tayside experience of programme budgeting and marginal analysis. *J Health Serv Res Policy* 1996;**1**:185–93.

91 Scott A, Donaldson A. Clinical and cost effectiveness issues in health needs assessment. In: Wright J, ed. *Health Needs Assessment in Practice.* London: BMJ Books, 1998.

92 Scott A, Henderson L. *Evaluating the Care of Stroke Patients in Nairn and Arderseir using Program Budgeting and Marginal Analysis.* Aberdeen: University of Aberdeen, Health Economics Research Unit, 1999.

93 Scott A, Wordsworth S, Donaldson C. *Using Economics in a Primary Care led NHS: Applying PBMA to GP Fundholding,* presented at Health Economists' Study Group. Brunel, 1996.

94 Scott A, Currie N, Donaldson C. Evaluating innovation in general practice: a pragmatic framework using programme budgeting and marginal analysis. *Fam Pract* 1998;**15**:216–22.

95 Scott A, Currie N, Wordsworth S, Donaldson C. *A PBMA of Asthma and Diabetes Care in the Nairn and Ardersier Total Fundholding Pilot Site. An Evidence-based Approach to Decision Making in Primary Care.* Aberdeen: Highland Health Board, 1998.

96 Scott A, Donaldson C, Scott S. Program budgeting and marginal analysis: pragmatism and policy (editorial). *J Health Serv Res Policy* 1999;**4**:1–2.

97 Scott S. *Programme Budgeting Marginal Analysis Exercise for General Surgery.* Paisley, Scotland: Argyll and Clyde Health Board, 1996.

98 Shiell A, Hall J. *Advancing Health in NSW: Planning in an Economic Framework.* Sydney: CHERE, 1993.

99 Spenceley S, Halma L. Improving surgical service utilization – An application of program budgeting and marginal analysis. *Ambulatory Surg* 2002;**10**:37–44.

100 Steele R, Gray A. Beyond the programme budget: Economics and resource planning in the NHS. *Hosp Health Serv Rev* 1980;**March**:96–101.

101 Steele R, Gray A. *The Identification of the Costs of Maternity Care: a Programme Approach to Health Service Expenditure.* Aberdeen: University of Aberdeen, Health Economics Research Unit, 1979.

102 Street A, Posnett J, Davis P. *Marginal Analysis of Dementia Services.* Report P2002a. York: Health Economics Consortium, University of York, 1995.

103 Twaddle S, McIlwaine G, Miller A. *Improving Gynaecology Services within Existing Resources: A Program Budgeting and Marginal Analysis Approach.* Glasgow: Scottish Forum for Public Health Medicine, 1994.

104 Twaddle S, Walker A. Programme budgeting and marginal analysis: application within programmes to assist purchasing in Greater Glasgow Health Board. *Health Policy* 1995;**33**:91–105.

105 Viney R, Haas M, Mooney G. Program budgeting and marginal analysis: a guide to resource allocation. *NSW Public Health Bull* 1995;**6**:29–32.

106 Viney R, Haas M, De Abreu LR. A practical approach to planning health services: using PBMA. *Aust Health Rev* 2000;**23**:10–19.

107 Wilson H, Scott S. PBMA – its role in the future purchasing arrangements for health care services. *Health Policy* 1995;**33**:157–60.

108 Wiseman V, Mooney G, Jan S. *Aboriginal and Torres Strait Islander Communities Setting their own Healthcare Priorities.* Sydney: University of Sydney, 1998.

109 Wiseman V, Mooney G, Stephenson J. *An Economic Approach to Priority Setting in Health Care.* Sydney: University of Sydney, 1998.

Appendix B: Details of PBMA exercises

Health authority	Dates	Micro or macro PB/MA	Specific programmes (if micro PBMA)	Comments on activity
United Kingdom				
Argyll and Clyde HB	1995	Micro and meso PBMA	General surgery	Activity continued
Ayrshire and Arran HB	Unknown	Unknown	Unknown	Details not known
Bury and Rochdale HA	Unknown	Unknown	Unknown	Details not known
Doncaster HA	1996–97	Micro MA	Maternity services	Work completed
Dumfries and Galloway HB	1997–98	Macro PBMA	–	Activity continued
Eastbourne HA	1993	Micro PB	Unknown	Unknown
East Kent HA	1996–99	Macro PB	Matrix across all HA expenditure	Ongoing
East Sussex HA	1991–96	Micro and macro PB with some MA	Matrix across all HA expenditure	One-off exercise
Fife HB	1994–97	Macro PB	–	Stopped due to change in NHS climate and expense of doing programme budget
Gloucestershire HA	Unknown	Unknown	Unknown	Unknown
Grampian HB	1974–76	Micro PBMA	Elderly	Unknown
Grampian HB	1976–77	Macro PB	–	Unknown
Grampian HB	1979	Micro PB	Maternity services	Unknown
Grampian HB	1980	Micro PBMA	Hospital pharmacy	Unknown
Grampian HB	1991	Micro MA	Dementia (elderly)	Activity continued
Grampian HB	1994–95	Micro PBMA	Maternity services	Activity continued
Grampian HB	1978–79	Meso PB	Matrix for lab services	Work completed
Grampian HB	1994–97	Micro and Macro PBMA	Various services	Stopped due to change in funding of health economics by board; political changes

(Continued)

(Continued)

Health authority	Dates	Micro or macro PB/MA	Specific programmes (if micro PBMA)	Comments on activity
Greater Glasgow HB	1993	Micro PBMA	Gynaecology	One-off exercise
Greater Glasgow HB	1998–99	Micro PB	Incontinence/ child health	Work completed
Greenwich HA	1994–96	Macro PB	Matrix across all HA expenditure	Stopped due to mergers of health authorities
Hastings HA	1991–96	Micro and macro PB with some MA	Matrix across all HA expenditure	One-off exercise
Highland HB	1996–97	Micro and macro PBMA	Physiotherapy; stroke diabetes; asthma	Micro tasks completed; macro possibly still ongoing
Lambeth, Southwark and Lewisham HA	1995–97	Micro and macro PBMA	CHD; maternal health; mental health	Each were one-off exercises; little success overall
Lanarkshire HB	1996–97	Micro PB	Unknown	Unknown
Leicester HA	1996–97	Micro MA	Diabetes	Work completed
Liverpool HA	1997–98	Micro PBMA	Asthma; stroke	Ongoing
Liverpool HA	1994	Micro PBMA	Mental health; heart disease	Activity continued
Lothian HB	1995–6	Micro PBMA	Child health services	Unlikely PBMA is still used
Nairn and Ardersier total fundholding pilot site	1994–6	Micro PBMA	Diabetes; asthma; stroke care	Activity continued
Newcastle District HA	1991–92	Macro PB	–	One-off exercise

(Continued)

(Continued)

Health authority	Dates	Micro or macro PB/MA	Specific programmes (if micro PBMA)	Comments on activity
Newcastle District HA	1994–98	Micro and macro PBMA	Heart disease; colorectal cancer	One-off exercise
Norfolk HA	1996–99	Micro and macro PBMA	Unknown	Ongoing
North-east Anglia HA	Unknown	Macro PB	Unknown	Unknown
North Yorkshire HA	Unknown	Unknown	Unknown	Unknown
Mid Glamorgan (Wales)	1993–94	Micro PBMA	Maternal/child; cerebral vascular disease; injuries; respiratory diseases; cancers; oral health; pain, discomfort and palliative care; physical and sensory disabilities; healthy living	One-off exercise
Oxford Region	1976–77	Macro PB	Matrix for geriatric, mental handicap, mental illness, maternity	Unknown
Rotherham HA	1994–95	Macro PB	–	Unknown
Seyton HA	1994	Micro PBMA	Mental health; heart disease	Activity continued
Scottish Audit Commission	1999	Macro PB	–	Considering using tool in audit of NHS
Scottish NHS	1991–96	Macro PB	Primary and secondary care	Used to determine resource shifts over time between sectors
Southampton HA	1994	Micro PB	Diagnosis related groupings	Unknown

(Continued)

(Continued)

Health authority	Dates	Micro or macro PB/MA	Specific programmes (if micro PBMA)	Comments on activity
South Thames Regional HA	Unknown	Unknown	Unknown	Unknown
St Helens and Knowsley HA	1994	Micro PBMA	Mental health; heart disease	Activity continued
Suffolk HA	1997–99	Micro and macro PB	Unknown	Ongoing
Sunderland HA	Unknown	Unknown	Unknown	Unknown
Tayside HB	1994–95	Micro PBMA	Child health	One-off exercise
Teesside HA	Unknown	Unknown	Unknown	Unknown
West Pennine HA	1995	Micro and macro PBMA	Mental health	Activity continued
Yorkshire Regional HA	Unknown	Unknown	Unknown	Unknown
Africa				
Ghana	1975–76	Macro PB	–	Unknown
Australia				
Cancer Network	1999/2000	Micro PBMA	Cancer services	Used DALYs as primary indicator of benefit
Central Coast AHS	1998	Micro PBMA	Mental health	Ongoing and spreading
Hunter AHS, New England AHS, Western Sydney AHS	1998–99	Micro PBMA	Dental services; diabetes	Ongoing
Macquarie Area Health Service	1997–98	Macro PBMA	–	Project done but still pervasive in culture
Mid Western Area Health Service	1998–99	Micro PBMA	Breast screening; alcohol and drug services rehabilitation	Ongoing (pilot projects)
South Australia Health Commission: application Flinders Medical Centre, Noarlunga	1997–98	Micro PBMA	Respiratory unit; surgical services; women's and babies; obstetrics,	Further in some cases

(Continued)

(Continued)

Health authority	Dates	Micro or macro PB/MA	Specific programmes (if micro PBMA)	Comments on activity
Hospital, Women's and Children's Hospital, North Western Adelaide Health Service, Royal Adelaide Hospital			surgery and cardiology; drug overdose	
South Australia Health Commission: North Metro CHS, Inner Southern CHS, Adelaide Central CHS, Noarlunga CHS	1996–97	Micro PBMA but more focus on MA	Men's and children's health; aboriginal health; women's health; non-intentional physical injury at home or leisure	Work completed
South Western Sydney AHS	1997–98	Micro PBMA	Coronary heart disease	
Territory Health Services	1998	Micro PBMA	Public Health Division	Work completed
Territory Health Services	1998	Micro PBMA	Public Health Division	Work completed
Torres Strait Islander District Health Service	1997–98	Micro MA	Community aboriginal services	Demonstration study but more to follow
Victoria	1999	Micro PBMA	Anti-smoking health promotion	Ongoing
Western Australia Health Department	1998	Micro PBMA	Cardiac services and rehabilitation	Ongoing
NSW Health: Central Coast AHS	1996–97	Micro PBMA	Dentistry	Activity continued
NSW Health: Greater Murray AHS	1996–97	Micro PBMA	Asthma	One-off exercise

(Continued)

(Continued)

Health authority	Dates	Micro or macro PB/MA	Specific programmes (if micro PBMA)	Comments on activity
NSW Health: Central Sydney AHS	1996–97	Micro PBMA	Child, adolescent and family community health	One-off exercise
South Australia Health Commission: North Metro CHS, Central Adelaide CHS, Noarlunga CHS	1996–97	Micro PBMA	Mental health services within community health sector	Unknown
New Zealand				
Central Regional Health Authority	1994–95	Macro PBMA	–	Stopped due to senior manage-ment
Southern and Midland health regions	1997/98	Micro PBMA	Respiratory disease	Informed business planning
Canada				
Calgary Health Region	2000	Micro PBMA	Paediatric transport	Successful one-off exercise
Calgary Health Region	2000	Micro PBMA	Infant cranial remodelling	Successful one-off exercise
Calgary Health Region	2000	Micro PBMA	Musculoskeletal health	Political issues prevented completion
Calgary Health Region	2001–02	Macro PBMA	Across all services	Activity continuing
Chinook Health Region	2000	Micro PBMA	Surgical services	Use ongoing

(Continued)

(Continued)

Health authority	Dates	Micro or macro PB/MA	Specific programmes (if micro PBMA)	Comments on activity
Chinook Health Region	2000	Micro PBMA	Rural chronic disease	Use ongoing
Headwaters Health Authority	2000	Micro PBMA	Surgical services	Successful one-off exercise
Headwaters Health Authority	2000	Micro PBMA	Long-term care services	Successful one-off exercise

HB, health board; HA, health authority; AHS, area health service; CHS, community health service; PB/MA, programme budgeting/marginal analysis; DALY, disability adjusted life year

7: PBMA case studies from the UK and Canada

Introduction

In this chapter two programme budgeting and marginal analysis (PBMA) case studies are presented which serve to exemplify many of the points made in the previous chapters. These case studies were selected to represent different levels of decision making in health organisations:

- meso – across programmes but still within a given service area
- macro – across programmes or portfolios within a single health organisation.

Although not presented here, one could also imagine an application of PBMA at a micro level, within specific programmes of care. Emphasis is given to how the multitude of inputs into decision making are incorporated into PBMA exercises (see Figure 5.1). Further, key "lessons learned", as presented in Chapter 5, will become more apparent, and a link to the Accountability for Reasonableness framework, outlined in Chapter 3, is also made. Of course, PBMA cannot meet every challenge faced by decision makers. One problem is that expectations of managers embarking on priority setting exercises are often quite high. Thus, this chapter also serves to highlight the limitations of PBMA more generally.

Meso PBMA: UK

Context

An example of a meso level PBMA study is from the Tayside Health Board,[1] which is based in the north-east of Scotland. It has a mixed urban–rural population of approximately 300 000, and its main city is Dundee. In the mid-1990s, the Health Board was seeking to plan child health services over the forthcoming 10-year period. The consultant in public health in charge of the review wanted to take a different approach to needs assessment by matching benefits produced by interventions to their costs, rather than relying on estimates of burden of illness. Because the consultant wanted to use an economic approach, he contacted the Health Economics Research Unit at the University of Aberdeen about providing consultancy services for the review.

In determining purchasing priorities in child health, decision makers and researchers constructed a strategic framework for incorporating data and viewpoints from numerous sources. It was recognised that not having objective and empirical evidence on health gain made assessing margins for change based on a marginal cost/ benefit framework very difficult. Thus, a pragmatic position was taken, as decision makers acknowledged that decisions still had to be made in lieu of detailed, research-based data. Their response was to utilise information from a number of difference sources including: an epidemiology-based needs assessment; national and local policy documents; consumer/public views; health professional views; a programme budget matrix; and effectiveness and cost-effectiveness research evidence.

Process used

The aim of the PBMA exercise was to develop clearly identifiable priorities for purchasing in the Health Board over the next 10 years. A needs assessment was first conducted to compile a health profile for the children within the Board, focusing in particular on key causes of mortality and morbidity. Policy documents were also reviewed to determine both national and regional objectives. As well, a programme budget was derived, containing activity and cost data for 10 broad service categories, split by various settings in which the services might be delivered – for example, one cell in the matrix was for inpatient general paediatrics, while another was for outpatient child psychiatry. The programme budget helped to define child health services and identify possible areas for changing service provision.

Views of health professionals were included through a two-staged approach. First, a multidisciplinary professional advisory panel was formed. Members were asked to generate up to 10 potential areas for service development, or investment, and 10 areas for resource release. The panel was also asked to justify their choices and specify projected health gains from the proposed changes. The second stage involved a mail-out survey of health professionals working with children. Upon reviewing the needs assessment findings and the programme budget, this broader group was asked to rank 10 areas for service development and 10 areas for resource release, from the services previously identified by the advisory panel, again on the basis of expected health gain.

Following this, a focus group of parents of children with health problems was established, as was an advertised phone-in over a 24-day period. Suggestions for improvement of services were noted and ranked according to frequency of report. Finally, a literature review was conducted for four specific areas identified by parents and providers as candidates for service development or resource release.

Process results

The 10 areas for development and resource release areas are displayed in Table 7.1, with strategy recommendations made to the Health Board. A simple point-scoring scheme was used whereby an option was given 10 points if ranked first, nine if second and so on. These points were then summed across respondents. Costs were assessed later, by examining the literature and local data. Areas for resource release were those that would result in little or no loss of benefit. The released resources were to be reinvested in service developments, thereby resulting in more benefits to the community as a whole from the total resources spent on child health services.

Lessons learned

There were several identified strengths of this exercise, including the fact that a consensus view of common priorities was able to emerge between providers and the public. Weaknesses of the study included the extent to which the formation of potential areas of investment and disinvestment was subjective and a lack of broad representation from the

Table 7.1 Tayside PBMA: suggested areas for service development and resource release ranked by frequency with which option was mentioned

Rank	Service development area	Score	Rank	Resource release area	Score
1	Children with special needs	866	1	School health service	1323
2	Community liaison officer	702	2	Health visitors	568
3	Respite care	653	3	Child development centre	527
4	Child protection	456	4	Child protection	459
5	Physiotherapy	421	5	Respite care	433
6	Services for adolescents	416	6	DRI – Ninewells	419
7	Day patient care	404	7	Hospital bed numbers	412
8	Health visitors	274	8	Immunisation (routine)	346
9	Child development centre	268	9	Management	323
10	School health service	222	10	Developmental screening	320

DRI, Dundee Royal Infirmary

community. In addition, the impact of each different source of information in the process was difficult to identify, although it was believed that the evidence from the literature review was least useful due to the lack of studies relevant to the local context and the paucity of costing data.

Nonetheless, despite a lack of "hard and fast" data supporting specific changes, the core team was able to pragmatically assess options for change, making judgements on the marginal costs and benefits of the services under consideration. While the priority setting process has to be recognised as partially a political one, PBMA clearly provides a forum through which evidence can be considered and decisions made.

It can also be observed that there is a discrepancy between the theoretical concept of the margin and the practise of PBMA. In principle, it is appropriate to think at the margin and attempt to identify the costs and benefits of changes in service provision. Indeed, in this example, this thinking was clearly present through the identification of potential boundaries where allocation of resources could be shifted to improve the overall health of the population. In practice, though, an approach was taken which included multiple sources, some guesswork, particularly for activity and cost data in the programme budget and, to a lesser extent, in the marginal analysis, and reliance on expert and community opinion. In the end, through this strategic approach to priority setting in Tayside, it was thought that a more rational and efficient allocation of resources would result.

Macro PBMA: Canada

Context

The Calgary Health Region (CHR) is an integrated, primarily urban health authority in southern Alberta which provides services across the continuum of care, from community health services to acute tertiary care. Its structure has seven Executive Director/Medical Director (ED/MD) pairs, each overseeing one major portfolio (i.e. medicine, surgery, community services, health promotion/prevention, children and women's health, and mental health), and who comprise the senior management team in the Region. At the time of the PBMA application, the Health Region was serving just under 1 million people, and the annual operating budget of the CHR was approximately Can$1.5 billion. As with most Canadian jurisdictions, the majority of physician reimbursement falls outside this budget, as it is paid directly from a separate "provincial pool" on a fee-for-service basis.

Process used

The CHR's short-term goal with this project was to aid in the development of the 2002/2003 budget across all seven major service portfolios. The longer term goal was to develop an explicit priority setting process that could be used annually as part of the business planning/budgeting cycle. The project was based on a form of social research called participatory action research, which has as its primary aim to instil change within an organisation. At the core of the process was an advisory panel which was comprised of the senior management team of the Health Region. This multidisciplinary group of clinicians, administrators and other financial personnel were charged with developing a list of service growth investment options, as in question 3 in Box 4.1, and, in order to fund these investments, lists of efficiency/productivity and service reduction options (questions 4 and 5 in Box 4.1). The panel then assessed the various options and made resource reallocation recommendations, based on a set of pre-defined, locally generated criteria. The step by step process is outlined in Box 7.1.[2]

Process results

Resources released through revenue generation and efficiency/productivity gains were directly shifted into areas for service growth, or other identified needs such as the projected deficit. As this process only enabled some of the service growth options to be funded, service reduction options were then ranked by the advisory panel alongside of the remaining service growth investment options. This ranking was done through a multi-voting, consensus process, with advisory panel members having the opportunity to provide rationale for items from their own portfolio. All members were given a set amount of votes with which to rank the options under consideration. Scores were tallied with those items achieving the most points being taken as highest priority. The criteria on which the decisions were based are given in Box 7.2; these were developed through limited community consultation, and were refined by advisory panel members.

In the end, approximately Can$45 million was released through efficiency gains and service reductions. Of this, about Can$42 million was allocated to the deficit, while the

Box 7.1 Prioritisation process in the CHR

Step 1: Portfolios identify service growth investment initiatives

- Each portfolio to rank their options and maintain "working list" of options

Step 2: Service growth investments identified and taken to regional table

- (a) ED/MDs discuss investment options with all relevant stakeholders within their portfolio including physician leaders
- (b) Top service growth items put forth regionally from each portfolio using a standardised business case format

Step 3: Identify portfolio efficiency/productivity opportunities

- Minimum per cent required based on annual regional targets
- One page standardised business case submitted centrally
- Use incentive plan to achieve targets as required
- Opportunities peer reviewed by senior management to ensure options are reasonable/achievable, with resubmission if rejected

Step 4: Identify service reduction opportunities

- Per cent required based on regional parameters
- One page standardised business case submitted centrally
- Use incentive plan to achieve targets as required
- Opportunities peer reviewed by senior management to ensure options are reasonable/achievable, with resubmission if rejected

Step 5: Decisions on shifting resources released from efficiency/productivity opportunities (from step 3) to growth areas, deficit or other use

Step 6: Develop a combined ranking of investments (from step 2) and service reduction options (from step 4) based on pre-defined criteria

- Multi-voting process used to reach consensus
- One list of service growth and reduction options formed; reallocation decisions from lower ranked disinvestments to higher ranked investments
- Capital items affecting operations ranked by ED/MDs, in addition to capital items already identified through operational prioritisation process

Step 7: Within portfolio validity check on reallocations with managers and physician leaders, and consultation with other stakeholders (for example human resources, IT)

(Continued)

Box 7.1 (continued)

Step 8: Recommendations to Executive and Board for final decisions as required

Step 9: Non-funded investments return to portfolios for potential funding through the incentive reinvestment process (or other internal reallocation)

- Central investment and disinvestment lists maintained; updated quarterly
- New growth, efficiency and service reduction proposals reviewed, with process recommencing from step 1 above

CHR, Calgary Health Region; ED/MD, Executive Director/Medical Director

Box 7.2 Prioritisation criteria*

1 Access/capacity
Improve access for pressure areas

2 Appropriateness
Enables shifts to services to more appropriate, lower cost settings

3 Sustainability/cost-effectiveness
Supports short- and long-term sustainability
Assists in avoiding tangible costs

4 System integration
Reduces service fragmentation
Supports best use of all elements of the health system

5 Clinical/population health effectiveness
Supports focused care for service populations
Improves clinical effectiveness

*Other health organisations may develop their own criteria.

remainder was available for additional reinvestment to service growth items, on top of about Can$12 million initially earmarked to service growth items at the outset of the process. An additional Can$1 million was released through service reduction, with those resources being made available for further investment in service growth areas as described above. Such large scale reallocations based on a marginal analysis type approach have not previously been reported in the literature.

Table 7.2 Lessons learned from CHR macro-level PBMA process

Comments from decision makers	Potential response from decision makers
Public involvement is important, but may not be best used in making allocation decisions between specific services	Input of public can come through contributions to the criteria and principles on which specific decisions are made, as well as in providing information on weighting individual criteria
There is a perception that members of the public do not accept the notion of resource scarcity	Education is required to ensure the public recognises that every day in healthcare decision makers ration services
Physicians are often ostracised from, or at least not fully integrated with, priority setting activity	Clinical expertise must be drawn into the priority setting process, in part through criteria development and in part through presenting relevant evidence
Comparison of disparate treatment groups and reallocation between different services is challenging	Pragmatic assessment of disparate groups based on pre-defined, locally generated criteria using a multidisciplinary advisory panel is feasible
Criteria on which priority setting activity is based are dynamic	Local surveys with decision makers, physicians and the public should be conducted regularly to identify criteria weighting and to determine whether new criteria have become relevant
Evidence is often unavailable or not used, resulting in a politically driven process that is open to "trumping" by senior executives and board members	Explicit, transparent processes for priority setting and resource allocation, which draw in local data and evidence from the literature, should be used, thereby providing less opportunity for protest and trumping
Development of an informed, evidence-based priority setting process takes time	Iterative development, with decision makers willing to take a longer term view on building a truly representative process key
The process itself can be overrun by "crisis" decision making	Proper planning of the budgeting/business planning cycle is required, including a timeline to achieve key milestones

(Continued)

Table 7.2 (Continued)

Comments from decision makers	Potential response from decision makers
Investment in longer term innovation is unlikely to occur with the usual focus on short term planning	Taking a portfolio analysis approach to investment, alongside of the PBMA approach, with allocation in "slow and steady" and perceived higher risk services should result in greater health gains overall
Processes of reallocation can be threatened because of a perception of "winners" and "losers"	Decision makers can be encouraged to take a genuine population health perspective, particularly if part of an "integrated" health organisation spanning the continuum of care

Lessons learned

Following implementation of PBMA at this macro level, a number of issues were identified through follow up interviews and focus group activity with senior managers and clinicians in the CHR. These are presented in Table 7.2, and highlight a number of lessons learned through this activity.

Link to ethical framework

As discussed in Chapter 1, economics is of course not the only discipline which can inform priority setting activity. While the PBMA approach, through the use of an advisory panel, allows for a broad set of criteria to be considered in the decision making process, it may be that other disciplines need to be more explicitly drawn upon. In conjunction with researchers at the University of Toronto,* the macro level PBMA application in the CHR was evaluated against the four main conditions which comprise the Accountability for Reasonableness framework, as given in Table 3.1. Highlighted in Table 7.3 are a number of relevant observations made by CHR decision makers.

---

*In particular, we would like to thank Dr Jennifer Gibson for her collaboration on this work.

Table 7.3 Accountability for Reasonableness and Macro level PBMA

Conditions	How PBMA in the CHR matched up
Publicity	• It was felt that improvements could be made so that the process itself was more widely understood within the health authority (internal publicity) • There was consensus that the process itself does not have to be made known to the public, but the decisions certainly would be public (as it will be seen what services are funded and what are not) (external publicity)
Relevance	• Rationales on which decisions were made were seen to be fair minded overall, however, better use of evidence was thought to be required, and more rigor in developing criteria on which decisions are made is needed, including greater public involvement • One means of ensuring better evidence to inform decision making would be even greater reliance on standardised business case template for all service growth and resource release items put forth
Appeals	• There was limited ability to appeal decisions once the voting process had proceeded, but it could be built in as a structured and explicit step in the PBMA model • It was also held that an appeal should not be allowed to proceed unless it was clear that new evidence became available to further inform the initial decision, and that distinctions should be made between an appeal of the process and an appeal of the decision
Enforcement	• Peer review by the senior management team was seen as a sound strategy for ensuring that realistic items were put forth on the growth and resource release lists, and that ultimately the "right" decisions were made • Longer term follow up and tracking of outcomes of reallocation decisions were seen as an important aspects of the process

More generally, those senior managers and clinicians interviewed in the CHR held that transparency of the process could be improved through ensuring adequate time is built in to enable dissemination within the organisation regarding the process being used, as well as to provide more information on the resulting recommendations. It was also held that both physicians and the public could be tapped into more explicitly for input into criteria development, on which the decision makers would base specific funding decisions.

In terms of fairness, the decision makers felt strongly that cross-portfolio comparison of disparate treatment groups was a necessary part of their jobs, and indeed could be conducted through pragmatic weighing out of relative value based on a set of underlying criteria. Despite not having a "common metric" to provide a specific quantitative assessment of the value of resource release proposals vis-à-vis service growth items, the advisory panel was able to make the necessary comparisons and resulting funding decisions. This notion is picked up on again in Chapter 10.

Summary

In some ways, the two examples used to illustrate the PBMA framework may not be that different from current practices elsewhere, except that with PBMA the decision making process, including the values and criteria on which decisions are based, is made explicit. In introducing an explicit approach to priority setting, the starting place is acceptance of scarcity and thus recognition of the need for reallocation to arrive at an optimally allocated set of resources. That said, this type of approach is not without challenges, and thus the next five chapters attempt to outline some of the key issues and means of moving through these challenges in the complex world of healthcare decision making.

Finally, only with longer term follow up of population health indices might the true impact of priority setting activity as described be identified. Of course, due to the many influences on individual and population health, it may not be possible to fully measure the impact of an explicit, evidence-based priority setting process in this way. It would also be extremely difficult to make comparisons between use of a PBMA approach and "what would have been" if an explicit approach was not used. This emphasises the importance of follow up surveys with users of the process which can inform iteration over time. The PBMA approach is realistic and pragmatic, and to date has been well received by both administrators and clinicians in many of the health organisations internationally where it has been applied.

References

1 Ruta D, Donaldson C, Gilray I. Economics, public health and health care purchasing: the Tayside experience of programme budgeting and marginal analysis. *J Health Serv Res Policy* 1996;1:185–93.
2 Mitton C, McGregor J, Conroy M, Waddell C. Making choices in health care: the reality of scarcity. *Hosp Q* 2002;6:48–54.

Part 4: Challenges to explicit priority setting

8: The challenges of data and time

Introduction

In the previous chapters, the basic economic concepts on which a priority setting approach should rest were outlined. Based on this, a "way of thinking" which can aid decision makers in dividing up the limited resources available in health organisations was set out. One approach which operationalises the economic way of thinking, and which has been used in a number of countries, is programme budgeting and marginal analysis (PBMA). Two case studies were presented in Chapter 7 to provide the reader with details on how this approach can be used, at different levels within a health organisation. As mentioned, though, PBMA is not without its challenges; a number of commonly identified challenges to PBMA are listed below.

- The challenge of data – concern with availability of data, specifically in terms of having locally relevant information for the reallocation process.
- The challenge of time – the perceived resource intensiveness of PBMA.
- The challenge of disinvesting – how to identify and release resources to fund candidates for expansion.
- The challenge of forming a programme budget – including the effort required and the usefulness of this process.
- The challenge of measuring and valuing benefits – use of options such as quality adjusted life years, willingness-to-pay and conjoint analysis.
- The challenge of involving the public – who should be involved and how.
- The challenge of organisational behaviour – barriers in both the uptake of an explicit process for setting priorities and in carrying out specific recommendations for reallocation.

The above challenges can appear formidable and have led some researchers to reject the PBMA approach outright,[1] while to others, these challenges have resulted in creative responses.[2,3] In the end, the merit of an approach for priority setting should be judged on the extent to which real or perceived challenges can be overcome, and how a given approach compares to others. With that in mind, the first two challenges listed above are discussed in this chapter, and the remaining are addressed in Chapters 9 through 12. While the focus is on PBMA, it is the case that most of these issues must be addressed in some form when using any explicit, informed approach to priority setting in health care.

The challenge of data

A widely cited concern in healthcare priority setting has been over data.[4] In determining how best to use available resources, two sets of information are required: that on costs and that on benefits or outcomes. The main challenges in this respect have been in obtaining relevant costing information and obtaining outcomes data that are reliable and locally applicable.

Costs

On the cost side, challenges can arise both when developing and populating a programme budget, as well as in marginal analysis when the impact of resource reallocation is being examined. For the programme budget, in many health organisations, acquiring cost data in the acute sector has become relatively straightforward. However, there can be major problems with obtaining reliable cost data for community services. Often required is an estimation of costs in a specific jurisdiction which has to be obtained from elsewhere, such as national data sets containing average costs for the types of services in question. As well, prospective survey work may also be required to fill in some of the gaps. As is discussed further in Chapter 9, it may be that extra resources will be required to develop a programme budget, particularly if the priority setting exercise includes service areas outside of the acute sector. It should be noted, however, that programme budgeting is meant to be a broad brush planning tool, so that devoting too much time and effort to precision is not normally a good investment. In other words, estimates will generally suffice.

In terms of marginal analysis, an important aspect for costing is in distinguishing between marginal and average costs. Noting the sixth stool guaiac case presented in Chapter 2, a marginal cost is the change in cost arising from an increase or decrease of one unit in service provision, whereas an average cost is the total cost divided by the total output. Due to fixed costs,* the marginal savings associated with a hospital bed closure are usually much lower than the average cost per bed-day. In considering the optimal level of service provision, it is marginal costs that need to be examined. This is because they reflect the resource implications of a *change* in service provision. It is this notion of changing or shifting resources that is central to the economic concept of the margin. Initially, one may think marginal cost figures cannot be derived, as cost centres within hospitals are designed for accounting purposes in which average cost is the more important figure. However, with some estimations marginal costs can be calculated.

For example, let us examine the issue of bed-day savings more closely. If a proposed disinvestment is to close five beds on a 20-bed ward, one would want to estimate all variable costs effected by this change, including things like nursing time, physician time, pharmaceuticals, kitchen staff and food consumption. In contrast, fixed costs such as those associated with general hospital administration, or resources tied up in capital infrastructure, would not be considered here. So, say a quarter of the beds on a given ward were closed, and this results in an estimated 20% of nursing time being saved. If there were five nurses on the ward previously, one of those nurses could now be cut back or redeployed. The cost of employing this nurse, available in the accounting department, could be used to calculate the savings in nurse time through the closure of the five beds. This type of analysis could also be

---

*Fixed costs are those which do not vary with the level of service provided (at least in the short or medium term).

done for each of the other variable resources. The key point is to recognise the type of costing required, and to focus on the impact of changes in resources. It is better to have a rough estimate of the right cost than a precise estimate of the wrong cost. Where the latter is the average cost a precise estimate is likely to be inappropriate for the purposes of the marginal analysis.

By making reasonable assumptions about what would be fixed and what would vary in different circumstances, as illustrated above, estimates on marginal costs can be obtained. In order to determine the robustness of the resource impact, some form of sensitivity analysis can also be used in the marginal analysis activity.[5] It is also useful to point out that the time frame is relevant. Over a longer period of time, more resources become variable, and marginal and average costs converge. A good example is an assumption that a hospital structure is fixed for most short and medium term analyses, but in considering a longer time horizon, it is conceivable that the building will be demolished. In this case, the resources tied up in the building become variable. This issue might actually arise in examining, say over a 20-year time period, the releasing of resources in acute settings for reinvestment in health promoting activity through community-based programmes. Importantly, the aim is in determining estimates for amounts of resources at the margin which could be taken from one area and shifted into services elsewhere.

Benefits

Shifting to outcomes, the main challenges for priority setting activity are a lack of data, or, if outcome data are available, their lack of local applicability. The key realisation here, though, is that regardless of whether an explicit approach to priority setting is being used, decisions have to be made in the face of the data that are available. Thus the challenge is not so much with a lack of data *per se*, but rather in how best to make decisions when detailed information on outcomes is not available. In fact, Cohen[2] argues that much can be achieved when only crude data are available.

At the outset, it is useful to remember that even if valid and reliable data are available, subjectivity still plays a role in the assessment of that data. When local data are not available, greater emphasis can be placed on the "expert" opinions of the decision makers. In some PBMA exercises, major emphasis has been placed on "hard and fast" evidence,[6] whereas in other cases, evidence from different sources has been pragmatically assessed, with greater emphasis on the opinions of those on the advisory panel.[7] Here the simple guide is about the cost of better data against the value added by these data. Clearly one wants to use evidence but the concept of best evidence is one that is subject to costs and benefits just as is the case with the production of other outputs. Further, interpretation of evidence and the values used in reaching decisions can often be at least as important as the evidence itself.

The issue of the application of evidence at the policy level has arisen in studies in the UK in regard to both decision making[8,9] and funding processes.[10] The question really is how can evidence be best used in decision making to support priority setting activity. Traditionally, researchers have held that well-designed randomised controlled trials (RCTs) are the gold standard. However, a strong case has been made that research should be designed and conducted with the context of the question in mind, and in many cases, an RCT will actually not be the ideal means to produce the "right" response.[11]

In fact, there is a growing recognition within the evidence-based medicine movement that evidence in different forms should be supported, and "softer" forms of evidence can be just as valuable in determining priorities. Such softer forms of evidence include qualitative data, non-randomised trials, information from other jurisdictions, and, as already discussed, the "expert" opinions of relevant stakeholders. One must be cognizant, however, that with greater reliance on pragmatic assessment of options, group dynamics will likely play a greater role in dictating final recommendations. Just as Kitson *et al.* argue that the successful implementation of research in practice is based in part on the nature of the evidence,[12] a key for the decision maker seems to be in recognising that evidence comes in different forms.[8]

In terms of the necessary skills to interpret research findings, it may well be useful for health organisations to invest in courses on research methods, focusing on skill building in areas such as literature review, study design and study biases. In addition, organisations should foster idea exchange between different organisational levels, and encourage dialogue between major service areas, particularly for macro-level priority setting processes. However, even the most skilled and informed personnel will be unable to apply evidence if the environment is not conducive to the thoughtful processing of evidence, in whatever form it comes. Thus, a response to the cultural challenge of a reactive environment would be to strike a priority setting team whose function would be to coordinate priority setting activity within the organisation, and importantly provide support in identification, and assistance in interpretation, of relevant decision making inputs, including evidence.[13]

The main point is to recognise that a lack of valid and reliable data does not have to be a barrier to the application of an explicit priority setting process. Perfection in data does not exist, and outcomes data should be viewed as only one input into the decision making process. If specific data are not available, a decision still has to be made. Decision makers should not be trapped in paralysis just because data are not available. Evidence, values and interpretation are always present although the mix will vary. The final mix will be a function of the costs and benefits of changing the existing decision base. In a given PBMA exercise, when relevant evidence is available it should be used, and when it is not, more reliance can be placed on "expert" opinions of the advisory panel.

The challenge of time

A further challenge to an explicit, informed approach to priority setting is the resource intensity of the activity. As has been exemplified in the previous chapters, priority setting which relies on a formal approach like PBMA has many components, with each having a potential draw on the health organisation's staffing. For example, decision makers often must rely on the interpretation and support of others. It is these additional resources that can quickly add up in terms of what is required to conduct the exercise. As well, the process may involve eliciting a range of views across the organisation or obtaining community input, which will cause the time to carry out the priority setting activity to increase.

Scarcity of time in decision making is a real issue in health care. Just how much time does a PBMA priority setting exercise take? Obviously, this will depend on the scale and scope of the exercise. Referring back to the macro-level work in the Calgary Health Region presented in Chapter 7, this exercise had an advisory panel of 20 senior management team members, who met for a total of about 40 hours over the course of a 6-month time frame. Financial and data analysts participated in the priority setting activity and provided support as part of their regular job duties. Micro and meso cases might take between 10 hours and 20 hours for the advisory panel meetings, with a range of 2–12 members, over periods of 3–12 months.

As reliance on locally-driven, primary research increases, timelines will extend. In the end, the time and effort for any given priority setting exercise will depend on multiple factors, including, amongst other things, the scope of the activity, the number of stakeholders involved, the complexity of the service areas under examination, the authority of and leadership on the advisory panel, and the support staff available.

One of the key advantages of PBMA cited in the literature is that the need for a fully fledged cost–benefit analysis is alleviated.[14] Advisory panel members in Alberta, interviewed following completion of specific PBMA exercises, have stated that the time demands required to complete the process were reasonable and that it fostered an evidence-based approach to decision making. In each instance, executives must weigh the costs and benefits of carrying out processes like PBMA. If significant engagement within an organisation is unlikely, and if in the end it is plausible that uptake of reallocation recommendations will not to be followed, then the organisation may be better served continuing with historically or politically driven priority setting processes. Careful selection of what information is needed in the decision making process is also important, as this will increase the resource intensiveness of the exercise.

Importantly, though, Mooney and Wiseman argue that while a given PBMA exercise can be labour intensive, healthcare managers should have no more important activity than that of setting priorities and allocating resources.[15] In fact, a broad group of Canadian decision makers recently put forth that priority setting is a very worthwhile activity, and one which should receive time even if other managerial activity is not pursued.[16] This issue is one of moving from crisis management to better informed, strategic planning and budgeting processes. It is also useful to examine the type of personnel who would be involved in the priority setting activity: the fire fighter-style managers may well be less likely to take up a PBMA process then the analyst-style managers. If priority setting is to be conducted in an area where there are mainly fire fighters, investing resources in an informed, explicit process may not be the best action at that time. Whether an approach like PBMA is adopted, or other explicit approaches to priority setting are developed, staff time will be required and each organisation will need to make its own assessment of the costs and benefits of this.

Conclusion

There is no doubt that explicit, informed approaches to priority setting in health care require both data and time. In thinking about data requirements, it is useful to note that decisions are made with limited data every day. Thus the challenge of having valid and reliable cost and outcomes data to support a priority setting process should not result in the rejection of forward thinking approaches. What is required is careful assessment of whether new approaches improve priority setting activity, to the extent that resources are allocated in a manner that results in local objectives being better met. Taking a pragmatic approach to decision making is arguably the way forward, so that data are used when available, but always with a mix of values and interpretation – the optimal mix depending on the costs and benefits in improved decision making.

In addition, the time requirements for explicit priority setting must be realistically weighed at the outset. In some instances, the incremental resources required to move into a PBMA-like approach may not be substantial as support personnel and decision makers alike will already be spending some time on priority setting and resource allocation activity. On the other hand, if a macro PBMA-like process is to be undertaken, significant engagement from both senior managers and key physician leaders must be realised, and the required commitment should not be viewed as insignificant.

No matter what approach is applied, the approach only provides a forum, and in the end, decision makers must grapple with information-limited decisions. There is no magic bullet for priority setting. As the health of the population is at stake, at least some time spent on setting priorities and allocating resources is probably a good thing. It is the opportunity cost of that time at the margin that must be weighed against the benefits of improved decision making for each priority setting environment.

References

1   Posnett J, Street A. Programme budgeting and marginal analysis: an approach to priority setting in need of refinement. *J Health Serv Res Policy* 1996;**1**:147–53.
2   Cohen D. Messages from Mid Glamorgan: a multi-programme experiment with marginal analysis. *Health Policy* 1995;**33**:147–55.
3   Peacock S. *An Evaluation of Program Budgeting and Marginal Analysis Applied in South Australian Hospitals.* Melbourne: Centre for Health Program Evaluation, Monash University, 1998.
4   Miller P, Parkin D, Lewis D, Gerard K. *Final Report of the Project "Developing Programme Budgeting and Marginal Analysis in Purchasing Organisations".* Newcastle: University of Newcastle upon Tyne, 1995.
5   Madden L, Hussey R, Mooney G, Church E. Public health and economics in tandem: programme budgeting, marginal analysis and priority setting in practice. *Health Policy* 1995;**33**:161–8.
6   Astley J, Wake-Dyster W. Evidence-based priority setting. *Aust Health Rev* 2001;**24**:32–9.
7   Ruta D, Donaldson C, Gilray I. Economics, public health and health care purchasing: the Tayside experience of programme budgeting and marginal analysis. *J Health Serv Res Policy* 1996;**1**:185–93.
8   Rosen R. Applying research to health care policy and practice: medical and managerial views on effectiveness and the role of research. *J Health Serv Res Policy* 2000;**5**:103–8
9   Newman M, Papadopoulos I, Sigsworth J. Barriers to evidence-based practice. *Intensive Crit Care Nurs* 1998;**14**:231–8
10   Dixon S, Booth A, Perrett K. The application of evidence-based priority setting in a District Health Authority. *J Public Health Med* 1997;**19**:307–12.
11   Birch S. Making the problem fit the solution: evidence based decision making and "dolly" economics. In: Donaldson C, Mugford M, Vale L, eds. *Evidence Based Health Economics: From Effectiveness to Efficiency in Systematic Review.* London: BMJ Books, 2002.
12   Kitson A, Harvey G, McCormack B. Enabling the implementation of evidence-based practice: a conceptual framework. *Quality Health Care* 1998;**7**:149–58.

13 Mitton C, Donaldson C. Setting priorities and allocating resources in health regions: lessons from a project evaluating program budgeting and marginal analysis (PBMA). *Health Policy* 2003;**64**:335–48.
14 Shiell A, Hall J. *Advancing Health in NSW: Planning in an Economic Framework*. Sydney: CHERE, 1993
15 Mooney G, Wiseman V. *Listening to the Bureaucrats to Establish Principles for Priority Setting*. Sydney, Australia: University of Sydney, 1999.
16 Mitton C, Donaldson C. *Priority Setting in health Care: From Research to Practice*. Edmonton: Alberta Heritage Foundation for Medical Research, 2002.

9: The challenges of disinvesting and the programme budget

Introduction

Two important issues are addressed in this chapter: identifying areas from which to release or disinvest resources, and the task of programme budgeting. The first issue is relevant if reallocation of the existing budget or a reduction in the budget is necessary. The second issue, that of programme budgeting, becomes important when wanting to map out current activity and expenditure to provide a broad picture of where one is before considering shifts in resources. How programme budgeting can be used, and indeed, whether this tool is even necessary, is examined.

The challenge of disinvesting

Setting the stage

A major challenge for an economic framework in the context of limited resources is that to fund proposals for expansions, unless there is an increase in the budget, resources have to be found within the existing budget. Several commentators would see this as the "Achilles heel" of a marginal analysis approach: either scarcity never bites or people are not willing to make the necessary trade-offs. In part, this criticism is justified, as rarely in health care are budgets truly fixed. Through government bailouts or revenue generation, health organisations will often have resource opportunities beyond what is initially budgeted. There is also, often to the detriment of marginal analysis activity, a culture in health care of expecting more resources rather than having to make trade-off decisions and reallocations.[1]

However, even if healthcare budgets are not always truly fixed, the principle of *re*allocation is still important. At some level, except where new monies are explicitly made available to fund additional service growth, existing services must be examined to try to release resources in order for investment to go ahead elsewhere. If operational efficiency can be improved (note question 4 in Box 4.1), resources can be shifted. The major hurdle, however, comes when decision makers want to fund more service growth than can be funded through new monies and improvements in operational efficiency. At this point, attention must be given to scaling back services which are providing positive benefits but where it is considered that there may be yet greater benefits to be had by shifting resources elsewhere (question 5 in Box 4.1). Thus, it is important for decision makers to weigh up the marginal benefit lost from scaling back a service with that of scaling up, or starting, some other service.

There are various ways of persuading managers and clinicians to think about the issue of disinvestment. These are discussed in the following subsections. While the methods discussed may seem simplistic, the importance of this issue should not be minimised, for if the challenge of releasing resource cannot be overcome, the essence of marginal analysis is lost. Further, any of the discussed strategies may also need to be tied to a set of incentives whereby individual programmes actually receive a certain percentage of every dollar released to reinvest in other opportunities in their own programme area. This is discussed in some detail in Chapter 12.

Thought experiments

One tool to aid in the process of identifying disinvestments is thought experiments. In these, groups are asked to think of what expansions they would set in place with some increment in total resources and what reductions they would suggest with an equivalent decrement in resources. Then, if total resources remained neutral, whether they in fact would still want to make these changes. A useful example of this, developed by David Cohen, a UK health economist, is to consider the following real-life scenario:

> The bread earner of the family comes home one night and she says to her husband and two children, "Guess what, today I got a letter from HR stating that my income will increase this year by 10%! So, what do we want to do that we couldn't do last year? Perhaps we should go to Disneyland this year, or maybe you want a new computer. Whatever you guys want I'm OK with it, you decide!"

> The next day, the woman comes home and says to her family, "Bad news! It turns out that I'm not as appreciated as I thought – I got a letter today stating that instead of a 10% raise, I'm actually getting a 10% reduction in salary. So, what can we now do without, that we had last year? Maybe you guys shouldn't enrol in hockey camp again this year, or perhaps we should cut out the annual trip to visit grandma and grandpa. What do you think?"

> On the third day, the woman comes home and says, "Blimey, everything was a big mix up. It turns out that my salary will neither decrease nor increase this year. Yup, it's staying the same. I guess the big question now is, do you still want to give up something from last year (e.g. the trip to the grandparents) so that we could do something else this year (e.g. go to Disneyland). If not, we are saying that we are currently using our income in the best way possible. If you do want to make some changes, though, it's no problem, it just means that we are agreeing that we could get more 'satisfaction' by doing some things differently."

One approach would be to pitch this type of thought experiment at a conceptual level at the outset of a priority setting application. The idea would be to use the thought experiment as a means of illustrating the economic principles of opportunity cost and the margin, and through this, to foster engagement with the group so that it is clear that not only is scarcity a reality, but that changing or shifting resources can be a positive action to take. Part of that shifting is ensuring that resource releases are identified because, as observed in the example about the family, if resources are not freed up in one area, the "wish list" or investment options simply cannot be funded in a resource neutral environment. Thought experiments could also be used in a more practical manner, for example as a guide to first work through identifying opportunities for investments, then disinvestments, then deciding if resources should be shifted assuming no changes in the overall budget.

Secret balloting

Practically, it would seem a key barrier for decision makers in identifying areas for resource release is in not wanting to be seen taking resources from someone else's programme area. One means of overcoming this problem is through using secret ballots. In a marginal analysis exercise, once all the proposed disinvestment items are listed by the advisory panel, secret balloting could be used to actually weigh disinvestment options against proposed service growth areas. In this way, choices between the proposed disinvestments and investments would be made anonymously. Not only does this serve to alleviate the social pressure faced by individuals on the advisory panel, but as well, it is a way to even out the playing field in instances where certain voices are rightly or wrongly given more weight. As well, the sophistication of the process could be improved by requiring each voter to briefly state on paper, again anonymously, why they voted as they did in the secret ballot, preferably with explicit reasoning based on any pre-defined decision making criteria.

One-on-one interviews

Another method that has been used in programme budgeting and marginal analysis (PBMA) applications, in order to generate options for both investment and disinvestment, is to have advisory panel members interviewed by a neutral person. This provides decision makers with the opportunity for considering options for change outside the group setting, in a structured format. In addition, the interviewer can provide an initial "validity check" of the proposed options. Suggested questions to guide the interview are found in Box 9.1. Of course, the actual amount used in the questions should be relevant for the scope of the exercise being conducted, but should be sufficient to challenge or stretch the panel members. Although potentially resource intensive, this can be a sound method for generating investment ideas and, more importantly, options for resource release.

Box 9.1 Suggested questions to guide the one-on-one interviews

If you were given $250 000 additional for your programme area, what specific services would you expand or introduce (and what are the resource implications and benefits of these expansions)?

If you were told that $250 000 would be taken away from your programme area, what specific services would be the first to go (and what are the resource implications and potential adverse effects)?

If you were told that $250 000 would be taken away from services *other than* in your programme area, but still within this health organisation, what areas or services would be the first to go (and what are the resource implications and potential adverse effects)?

The challenge of programme budgets

Setting the stage

One of the main questions raised about PBMA is whether programme budgeting is actually necessary. As noted in Chapter 5, the programme budget is a statement of how resources are currently used within or across programmes. Programme budgeting is perhaps best viewed as a framework for planning,[2] and can be thought of as the launching pad for marginal analysis. This tool provides a map of expenditure, or in some cases activity, but is not meant to provide a solution as to the best way forward. It gives information on how many resources are available and ways in which they are currently spent. In essence, programme budgeting provides information on the resources used – that is, the inputs – of a particular programme or set of programmes and relates this to the outputs achieved. As well, information on a population can be tracked in terms of various elements such as health status or socioeconomic status.

It is relevant to note that programme budgets are widely used in most business environments outside of health care. For example, a manufacturing company will constantly re-evaluate its "product portfolio" by analysis of product costs and profit margin. Discussions are then made to expand some product lines, delete others and create new ones all within an overall budget. Similarly, a services company will analyse their overall operating budget by type of service provided, such as design, planning, failure analysis, etc., against profit earned by each of those programmes. Resource shifting, or staff reassignment, will be made accordingly to maximise profits commensurate with corporate goals. This is in part the focus of "management accounting" as opposed to "financial accounting". Many texts are available on the subject for those who wish to probe deeper into the theory of the subject. The point to take here is that the programme budget provides the overall frame within which any changes to the current allocation can be made.

Examples of programme budgeting from Alberta

In order to illustrate more clearly what programme budgeting is, an example is provided here from Alberta, Canada. The Calgary Health Region, a largely urban health authority in southern Alberta, can be geographically split into six subregions, based on postal code. Through linking various components of the healthcare system, an overall picture of healthcare spending, in comparison to a health status measure, can be depicted (Table 9.1).

Total inpatient costs were derived by summing the cost assigned to every hospital episode for the fiscal year 1997/1998 in the region; total health care use includes inpatient, emergency, general practitioner and physician specialty costs. Potential years of life lost (PYLL) is a measure of the impact of various diseases on society, and highlights the loss to society as a result of early deaths.[3] PYLL was calculated here by dividing the total number of years of lost life due to all causes (relative to normal life expectancy) by the number of deaths, in each locality. This health status measure indicates the average number of premature years lost per death; a lower

Table 9.1 Healthcare spending and potential years of life lost (PYLL) by locality for 1997/1998 (CAN$)

Calgary by locality	Registry population	Average income	PYLL	Total inpatient use	Inpatient use per person	Total healthcare use	Total use per person
Northwest Calgary	206 247	$21 583	19.2	$68 807 886	$334	$134 959 233	$654
Northeast Calgary	203 643	$14 320	20.8	$70 062 092	$344	$142 786 175	$701
South Calgary	185 594	$23 636	18.1	$54 688 617	$295	$117 884 371	$635
West Calgary	123 336	$25 858	16.5	$51 175 499	$415	$99 768 159	$809
Central Calgary	69 398	$19 370	15.3	$36 008 620	$519	$63 427 579	$914
Outlying Communities*	43 785	$19 545	21.5	$18 842 086	$430	$44 351 074	$1013
Total Calgary	832 003	$20 975	19.5	$299 584 800	$360	$603 176 591	$725

*Postal codes representing rural communities which are included in this health region.

PYLL can be viewed as an indicator of a healthier and thus less "needy" locality.

It can be observed that, on a per capita basis, the Central and West localities have the lowest PYLL measures, i.e. the "best" health, and also have, respectively, the second and third most resources spent per head. It can also be seen that the Northeast has the second highest PYLL but only the fourth most resources spent. While these figures cannot inform how resources *should* be allocated, it is the case that depicting the information in this manner enables questions to be asked about the current mix of resources within the Region. Further analysis may reveal that the patterns observed in Table 9.1 are reasonable, or it may be that problems exist in the current spend. Either way, the programme budget provides a starting point for further examination of the data.

Prior to developing this programme budget, decision makers in Calgary stated an interest in knowing how resources were being spent in the Region according to geographical proximity. In other contexts, the relevant factor on which to split the data will be on age and in others on disease grouping or care setting.[4] The key is to depict the data in a manner which provides an "as-is" description of current expenditure, and through this, to identify if any issues "jump out" from the data, which might require further analysis.

In order to derive a programme budget, the activity and cost data must be available or made available either in administrative databases, or as discussed in Chapter 8, prospectively collected through survey work. It is to be noted however, that fine precision is not the aim with the programme budget – higher level costing at this stage will generally suffice. Finally, as already alluded to, the depiction of expenditure information often ends up posing more questions than answers. This is an important purpose of programme budgeting, as through examination of data in ways perhaps not previously considered, questions about potential areas of concern can be generated. Then, through marginal analysis, options for shifting resources can be explored.

Is the programme budget really necessary?

It has been argued that as marginal analysis is the key evaluative component of PBMA, the programme budgeting

Table 9.2 Reasons for and against programme budgeting

Reasons against programme budgeting	Reasons for programme budgeting
Activity and costing data may not be available, particularly for community services	No matter how few data exist, decisions still have to be made Desire for using programme budgets may drive data collection
Available data may not be wholly accurate	This is a broad brush planning tool; the aim is to paint a general picture of resource use
As it is not an evaluative tool, the information will often not be used	It is useful to know where one is prior to making recommendations for shifting resources around It is a flexible tool which can enhance accountability through comparing resource patters to specific objectives Comparison with historical patterns or other jurisdictions can also be made
The important aspect of PBMA is the marginal analysis	Prior knowledge of where the margins are may not exist, and thus there is a need to map this out with programme budgeting

step can simply be skipped over. In Table 9.2, points both for and against using programme budgets within the context of setting priorities are raised. Although there are several potential challenges with the development of programme budgets, in the end, programme budgeting is a tool which provides a framework through which questions can be asked and areas for further study can be highlighted.

A programme budget can point to possible problems in the allocation of resources over time, and can allow for comparison with stated regional or other provincial and federal health agendas or with the allocation of resources in other regions. As well, the programme budget can provide a broad overview of resource allocation patterns which otherwise may not be readily available in health organisations. Further, issues of equity can be highlighted as the programme budget indicates where and on whom resources are currently being spent. Finally, and perhaps most importantly, the programme budget makes the resource allocation process more explicit, and as such, can point to particular areas for more indepth evaluation with marginal analysis.[5]

References

1 Scott A, Donaldson C, Scott S. Program budgeting and marginal analysis: pragmatism and policy, (editorial). *J Health Serv Res Policy* 1999;**4**:1–2.
2 Mooney G, Russell E, Weir R. *Choices for Health Care: a Practical Introduction to the Economics of Health Provision.* London: Macmillan, 1986
3 Last, J. *A Dictionary of Epidemiology.* New York: Oxford University Press, 1995.
4 Miller P, Parkin D, Craig N, Lewis D, Gerard K. Less fog on the Tyne? Programme budgeting in Newcastle and North Tyneside. *Health Policy* 1997;**40**:217–29.
5 Cohen D. Messages from Mid Glamorgan: a multi-programme experiment with marginal analysis. *Health Policy* 1995;**33**:147–55.

10: The challenges of measuring and valuing benefits: economics-based methods

Introduction

Given the number of factors to be considered in healthcare decision making, composite measures of benefit may serve as useful aids in weighing up the various service and treatment options. The basic issue, in this respect, is how to measure the benefits of health care. In returning to the central concept of opportunity cost, an "economics-based" measure of benefit involves the notion of sacrifice. That is, something is not of value unless one is prepared to give up something else in order to obtain it. The maximum sacrifice one is prepared to make represents the value of the particular good under scrutiny.

The first part of this chapter builds on this notion of sacrifice by showing how it serves as a basis for a commonly applied measure of benefit in economic evaluation, the quality adjusted life year (QALY). Discussion of the QALY arose earlier, in Chapter 4, in the form of league tables, and thus the focus in this chapter is on the construction of the QALY measure itself. Also discussed are two measures which could potentially be used in priority setting: willingness-to-pay (WTP) and discrete choice experiments (DCEs). The basis of WTP and DCEs are described before providing examples, as was done for QALYs in Chapter 4, of how they have been used in decision making contexts. The relative merits of each measure are also discussed, along with what aspects of "benefit" are covered and their potential added-value to a marginal analysis process. For a more comprehensive description of these methods, the reader is referred elsewhere.[1,2]

Quality adjusted life years (QALYs)

Overview

The QALY is a health outcome measure which considers both quality and quantity of life over some period of time. The quantity component of the QALY is simply the number of life years under consideration. This can be the number of life years saved, which would be the extension of an individual's life, measured in years, due to a particular course of treatment. Alternatively, quantity of life can be a measure of a specific time span during an individual's life, say, when an individual has a non-life threatening illness which impacts their quality of life and lasts for some period of time.

The quality component of the QALY, or quality adjustment for each life year under consideration, can be derived through a number of different methods. In each case, a measure between 0 and 1 is derived, with 0 generally being equated with death and 1 with full health. Different states of health, lying between these two anchor states, are assigned scores between 0 and 1 depending on their severity. The methods for deriving these scores, often referred to as utilities or health state valuations, are described below.

Once an index or quality adjustment score has been obtained, the number of years under consideration is multiplied by the index score to derive the QALY. An illustration is provided in Figure 10.1, where, prior to a treatment for a specific condition, the mean QALY score for a group of patients was 0·6, which was calculated by taking the index score of 0·2 and multiplying it by the expected length (3 years) in that reduced quality state. Following treatment, this same group had a mean index score of 0·8 and would be expected to live in that state for 10 years. The difference in QALYs between the two scenarios is the QALY gain, which equals 7·4 in the example. That is, for these patients, on average, 7·4 QALYs would be added or gained by undergoing the given treatment.

Generic QALYs

There are two main types of QALYs: generic and condition specific. Generic QALYs can be applied to any group of interest

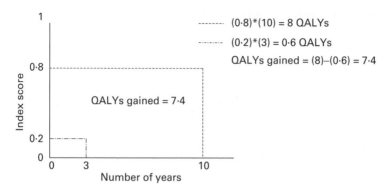

Figure 10.1 Diagrammatic illustration of QALYs

and are typically based on scores from the general public. Patients in a given study could be asked to complete a questionnaire in which they rate themselves in terms of different dimensions of health. The responses on these dimensions correspond to health states which have been scored, previously, by members of the general public. The scores, or utilities, corresponding to the health state indicated by the patients under study through the questionnaire, can then be multiplied by the relevant expected length of life to derive the QALY.

Generic QALYs are usually based on multi-attribute utility scales (MAUS), which are instruments for estimating health state values. The five most widely used MAUS are:

- Quality of well-being scale[3]
- Rosser's disability/distress classification[4]
- 15D[5]
- Health utility index versions one, two and three[6]
- Euroqol EQ-5D.[7]

Of these, the most common is the EQ-5D. The five dimensions of the EQ-5D are mobility, self-care, usual activities, pain/discomfort and anxiety/depression. Each dimension has three levels, as found in Box 10.1, thus enabling the EQ-5D to define 243 different health states. Adding two extra health states, unconscious and dead, yields 245 possible health state descriptions. The EQ-5D is designed to be administered in the form of a self-completed questionnaire. Subjects are asked to define their own health state in terms of the five dimensions and their levels, and then are asked to mark on a visual analogue scale how good or bad they think their current health is.

Box 10.1 Dimensions of the Euroqol EQ-5D

Mobility

- I have no problems in walking about
- I have some problems in walking about
- I am confined to bed

Self-care

- I have no problems with self-care
- I have some problems washing or dressing myself
- I am unable to wash or dress myself

Usual activities (for example work, study, housework, family or leisure activities)

- I have no problems with performing my usual activities
- I have some problems with performing my usual activities
- I am unable to perform my usual activities

Pain/discomfort

- I have no pain or discomfort
- I have moderate pain or discomfort
- I have extreme pain or discomfort

Anxiety/depression

- I am not anxious or depressed
- I am moderately anxious or depressed
- I am extremely anxious or depressed

Based on the time trade-off technique, described in the following subsection, a tariff of quality of life scores for each EQ-5D health state has been developed. The tariff was based on health state values elicited in a large scale survey undertaken in the UK,[8] and allows each of the EQ-5D health states, identifiable by a unique five-digit number corresponding to the levels for each of the five dimensions, to be converted into a score which can be used as the quality adjustment weight in the calculation of QALYs. Scores based on a North American sample have also been derived.[9]

In general, MAUS are relatively easy to conduct and often have low patient burden. However, the EQ-5D has been criticised for being too simplistic and insensitive to changes in health status.[10] Still, a recent review of the literature pertaining to the five main MAUS concluded that on the basis of a number of factors, such as practicality, reliability and various dimensions of validity, the EQ-5D and the Health Utilities Index should be the scales of choice.[11]

Condition-specific QALYs

For condition-specific QALYs, the health state descriptions provided to the subjects under study focus directly on the characteristics of the condition being evaluated. There are two main methods of generating condition-specific QALYs:

- standard gamble
- time trade-off.

The standard gamble is based directly on the axioms of standard utility theory and is the classic method of measuring preferences under uncertainty. The technique can be used to measure health state preferences for chronic and temporary health states. The discussion here focuses on the use of the technique to calculate QALYs for a chronic health state preferred to death.*

An example of the standard gamble is shown in Figure 10.2. To measure preferences for health state i, subjects are asked to choose between two alternatives. One offers the certain outcome of remaining in the chronic health state for the rest of one's life, whilst the other is a gamble representing a treatment with two possible outcomes. These two outcomes are to return to full health for the rest of one's life, with an associated probability P of occurring, or immediate death, which has a probability of occurrence of $1-P$. The probability P of a successful outcome is varied by an iterative process until the subject is indifferent, i.e. they cannot decide, between the gamble and the certainty. The probability at which the subject is indifferent is taken as the utility value of the health state, which can be used to calculate the QALY.

---

*For details of how the standard gamble can be applied to temporary health states and health states not preferred to death see Froberg and Kane,[12] Torrance,[13] or Johnston *et al.*[14]

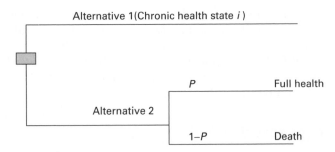

Figure 10.2 Standard gamble for a chronic health state preferred to death

Time trade-off was developed in the early 1970s as a substitute for the standard gamble technique.[15] The intention was to develop a technique specifically for use in health care, which gave the same or similar values as the standard gamble but which was easier for subjects to understand. Two important differences between time trade-off and the standard gamble should be noted. First, time trade-off does not have an axiomatic foundation, and second, subjects are asked to choose between two certain alternatives rather than between a certain outcome and a gamble. Like the standard gamble, time trade-off can be used to elicit health-state preferences for chronic and temporary health states that may or may not be preferred to death.

An example of the time trade-off approach for a chronic health state preferred to death is shown in Figure 10.3. Preferences for health state i are established by eliciting from subjects the number of years in full health (Z years) that is equivalent to spending the rest of their life (T years) in the chronic health state. The number of years in full health (Z) at which the subject is indifferent between the two alternatives is divided by T to derive the value of the health state, which can then be used to calculate the number of QALYs from the treatment in the same way as for the standard gamble.

Healthy year equivalents and QALYs

In recent years, an alternative to QALYs has been developed – the healthy year equivalent (HYE).[16] There is controversy

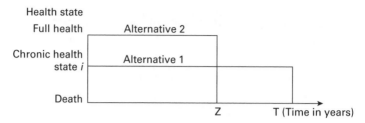

Figure 10.3 Time trade-off for a chronic health state preferred to death

within health economics as to the added value of HYEs over QALYs and the reader is referred to articles by the critics[17,18] and the advocates.[19,20]

One final thing to note is that none of these measures, and specific methods described to determine the measures, supply a "pure" indication of the value or utility of health. Different measures come up with different values because, to varying degrees, the scores obtained are contaminated by respondents' attitudes to time and risk.

Willingness to pay (WTP)

The most common method of measuring healthcare benefits in cost–benefit analysis is WTP. The principle of WTP is that the utility an individual gains from something is valued by the maximum amount that he or she would be willing to pay for that something. With this technique, individuals are given a description of a health state, or different types of health care, and are asked, hypothetically, what is the maximum amount of money that they would be willing to pay for that state or type of care. WTP can be used in the context of questions pertaining to both allocative and technical efficiency. An example is provided in Box 10.2.

The technique of WTP is often criticised for attempting to assign a monetary value to things that are considered by many to be incommensurate with monetary valuation, for example the environment or human life. However, it has to be remembered that such valuations are being made, often

Box 10.2 Closed-ended willingness to pay (WTP) survey question

Would you be willing to pay $2000 for treatment X? (A description and potential benefits of treatment X would be provided here)

YES_____   NO_____

implicitly, anyway. What is important is not the unit of value *per se*, but rather the notion of sacrifice embodied in the technique. In valuing a healthcare programme, it is difficult to ask respondents what services they would give up to have more of that programme. It is easier to ask individuals to state the maximum amount that they would be willing to pay for more of the programme and for some possible alternative uses of those resources. Thus, it is largely for convenience of comparison that money is the chosen numeraire.

One key advantage of WTP over other measures of benefit such as the QALY is that it provides the opportunity for individuals to value other potential benefits of health care beyond just health gain. One of the assumptions of QALYs is that the only benefit from health care is improvement in health-related quality of life. However, there is evidence that this is not always the case.[21] Other possible sources of benefit might include the provision of information (for example from screening), location (for example in maternity care), dignity (for example in long-term care), autonomy (for example in community care) and the process of care (for example invasive versus non-invasive interventions).

Depending upon the context of the evaluation, there are a number of different ways in which individuals can be asked about their WTP. These include out-of-pocket payments, one-off extra taxation payments, and payments for insurance. There are also a number of different ways of asking WTP questions. These include payment card questions, in which subjects are presented with a series of prompts from which to select a value, open-ended questions, in which respondents are asked to state their maximum WTP without prompting, and closed-ended questions, in which each respondent is presented with a WTP value and asked to indicate whether or not they would be prepared to pay that amount. All of these methods have advantages and disadvantages.[22]

Although WTP does define benefit more broadly than QALYs, a frequent criticism is that WTP is inevitably a function of ability to pay, which, it is argued, could have implications for equity. This can be dealt with, however, by weighting the WTP values. It can be noted that QALYs suffer from a similar problem but, as with WTP values, QALYs can also be weighted to reflect concerns such as severity of illness. These issues stem from the fact that all such measures are proxies for utility because utility itself cannot be measured directly.

Lastly, in cases where the total WTP elicited from users of a programme is greater than the programme cost, it may be tempting to conclude that such a programme is worthwhile. However, the opportunity cost context, especially in publicly funded healthcare systems, is one where resources for such a programme will have to come from some other use. Further, in determining "worthwhileness", the relevant set of values are those of the broader community, as opposed to the individual users of the service, as the question is one of allocative efficiency. That said, the WTP values of the users of the services being evaluated are still useful in this context. For instance, such values could indicate that the preferences of a minority group are particularly strong. If this strength of preference is not sufficient to outweigh that of the majority, such values may still indicate to the decision maker that providing both types of care being evaluated is the fairest option. Of course, it should be remembered that providing such choice may come at a substantial cost.

Discrete choice experiments (DCEs)

With DCEs, individuals are presented with hypothetical scenarios comprising different levels of various attributes and are asked to make pairwise choices between the scenarios,[23] an example of one such scenario being found in Figure 10.4. In this way, the relative importance of key attributes, vis-à-vis each other, can be identified. As well, the optimal way of providing a particular service, and the change in utility from moving from one type of service to another, can also be determined from the selections of the respondents. This technique can be used to address questions of technical or

Choice 1	Clinic A	Clinic B
Attitudes of staff towards you	Good	Good
Chance of taking home a baby	25%	25%
Continuity of contract with same staff	No	Yes
Time on waiting list for IVF attempt	18 months	18 months
Cost to you of IVF attempt	$1500	$3000
Follow-up support	No	No

	Prefer clinic A	Prefer clinic B
Which clinic would you prefer (tick only one box)		

Figure 10.4 Example of a discrete choice experiment (DCE) survey question

allocative efficiency, and has the potential to elicit not only patient preferences, but can also be used, as is shown below, in priority setting endeavours to determine relative values of services from the perspective of the provider or manager.

As with WTP, DCEs also incorporate the concept of opportunity cost, as respondents are asked to make explicit trade-offs in a series of choices between two scenarios. In addition, the intensity of preferences is derived, and unlike WTP, the health and non-health attributes are broken down, enabling weightings for particular attributes to be determined. Health and non-health attributes are also considered in WTP, but in this case the overall state is valued as a whole. That is, preferences for the individual components of the state are not able to be disaggregated from the overall state in WTP exercises. If DCEs are to be used to address allocative issues, involving comparisons of disparate alternatives, a set of attributes which can be used to describe all such alternatives has to be agreed upon.

There are two main limitations with DCEs.[24] First, it is not clear if the responses to hypothetical scenarios are different to those which would be elicited if the individual was actually faced with the same choice in "real life". This potential limitation also exists for WTP and QALYs, and arises in particular when questions of allocative efficiency are being addressed. This is because, as alluded to above, it is better for responses in allocative scenarios to come from community members at large, as in order to fund the option under consideration, resources would have to be allocated at the expense of doing something else. Thus, a broader perspective than the individual patients under question is appropriate. In these instances, hypothetical scenarios are the only way to present the problem and elicit a valuation. However, when questions of technical efficiency arise, it is more appropriate to elicit preferences from individuals with the condition, and thus alleviate the need for hypothetical scenarios, as the respondents are the ones actually faced with the treatment in question.

A second limitation of DCEs is that if cost is included as an attribute, the respondents may not be comfortable with the implications of the study and thus may not answer honestly, or may refuse to answer altogether. At present, more research is required into the validity of the responses when various attributes are included in the scenario provided to the respondent. This challenge could also potentially arise with WTP in the form of a social desirability bias, whereby individuals may overvalue a particular condition because they might perceive the condition to be of importance to society, regardless of that individual's own preferences.[25]

Using WTP and DCE data
in healthcare decision making

A recent example of using WTP to aid priority setting was an evaluation of public sector healthcare programmes in northern Norway.[26] Members of the public were asked their WTP in extra taxation for each of the following:

- the introduction of a helicopter ambulance service to serve remote communities
- an expansion in the number of heart operations performed
- an expansion in the number of hip operations performed.

Subjects were presented with detailed descriptions of the programmes and were told that only one could be implemented. They were also asked to state the reasons for their WTP responses. The study showed that WTP for hearts and the helicopter were about equal on average (each just over NOK300 (NOK, Norwegian kroner)) and that WTP for each of these was significantly different from the WTP expressed for hips (NOK230). The orderings one would establish from these results is different from what would be gained from calculations of QALY gains, which would rank hips highest. The results also indicated that individuals were concerned with more than just health gain from health care. This was shown by subjects' concern for other people's access to care. It appeared that subjects were prepared to express this concern in the values that they ascribed to the ambulance service vis-à-vis the other programmes.

As the first survey of its kind, one would not place too much store in the actual results; for example, the WTP questions relating to hips were always asked after those for hearts and helicopters, which may have deflated their valuations. Rather, the value of the work is more in the demonstration of people's willingness to participate in such surveys and the potential of the method to inform real-world decision making in health care. This research project spawned a major project, EuroWill, funded by the European Commission, to investigate various methodological issues associated with using WTP to value disparate healthcare alternatives.[27-30]

The use of WTP can also be used to address narrower questions. A recent example of this was in a study in the UK in which the relative benefits of two alternative locations for delivery of a baby were evaluated.[31] Using the results from a previously completed randomised trial, pregnant women were given descriptions of care in midwife-managed units and in traditional labour wards. They were asked for their preference for one over the other and then were asked about their maximum WTP to have their preferred rather than their less-preferred option. The results displayed a clear preference for the midwife-managed unit. However, the midwife-managed unit was also more costly than the labour ward. From a decision maker's perspective, a judgement would thus be required to determine if the extra benefit gained would be worth the extra cost. As the extra resources have to come from some other (presumably beneficial) service, more information about the alternative uses of those resources would be necessary before an informed funding decision can be made.

In terms of DCEs, a recent exercise was conducted as part of a priority setting process in Scotland.[32] This study set out to use the DCE approach to aid in the ranking of clinical service development proposals for a large acute teaching hospital. The hospital trust wanted to determine how to get as much benefit as possible in return from a series of investment proposals, with the benefit reflecting the preferences of the consultants working in the hospital. The first part of the exercise had about 130 consultants carry out a DCE, whereby each individual had to make selections between hypothetical pairwise scenarios, with the levels of the attributes varying between scenarios. The dimensions of benefit included were:

- level of evidence of clinical effectiveness
- size of health gain
- contribution to professional development
- contribution to education training and research
- match with local or national strategy areas.

Once the preferences of the consultants were obtained, a regression analysis was conducted to determine the relative weighting of each dimension of benefit.

The second part of the exercise had the clinical directors from across the hospital rate their own clinical service proposals on the same benefit dimensions used in the first part of the exercise. For example, a given service proposal may have been rated as having medium level of evidence of effectiveness, large health gain, no change in contribution to professional development, contribution to education and research but not training, and to effect local but not national strategies. Each of these proposals were then weighted according to the information provided by the consultants, and in the end, a utility ranking of all the proposals was compiled. The clinical directors also provided information on the cost of each proposal, and thus a cost per unit of benefit listing was also produced.

Most significantly, this exercise indicates very clearly that DCEs can be used in an actual priority setting process. As a limited amount of new monies was made available for growth options, the rankings provided an indication of how the most benefit could be derived. Although not done in this example, such an approach could also be used to rank potential service disinvestments, thereby providing information on where resources could be released to invest in the growth options.

From these examples, it can be seen that both WTP and DCEs can be used directly to aid priority setting activity in health care. As decision makers assess service growth, disinvestments and reallocation options, formalising benefit measurement with these techniques may prove useful. This can take the form of eliciting preferences from the community, which can feed into a priority setting process, or in directly assisting in the ranking of options for priority setting. Similarly, QALYs may provide additional information that is of use to decision makers, although as it is a more limited measure of benefit, it should be used at a minimum along side of other benefit measures to ensure that important aspects of benefit are not being lost.

Summary

All of the techniques discussed in this chapter are important economic contributions to measuring both health and non-health benefit arising from health services. In and of themselves, these techniques can be used to inform specific decisions about how best to spend limited resources. They can also be used to feed into a marginal analysis priority setting process. Although there are challenges in so doing, including the resource intensiveness and expertise required, making strides in this direction would shore up the evidence base on which decisions are made. This, in itself, is likely to lead to improved priority setting and better resource allocations.

References

1 Drummond M, O'Brien B, Stoddart G, Torrance G. *Methods for the Economic Evaluation of Health Care Programmes*. Oxford: Oxford University Press, 1997.
2 Nord E. *Cost-Value Analysis in Health Care*. Cambridge: Cambridge University Press, 1999.
3 Kaplan RM, Bush JW, Berry CC. Health status: types of validity and the index of well-being. *Health Serv Res* 1976;11:478–507.

4   Rosser R, Kind P. A scale of valuations of states of illness: is there a social consensus? *Int J Epidemiol* 1978;**7**:347–58.

5   Sintonen H, Pekurinen M. A fifteen-dimensional measure of health-related quality of life (15D) and its applications. In: Walker SR, Rosser RM, eds. *Quality of Life Assessment: Key Issues in the 1990s*. London: Kluwer Academic Publishers,1993:185–95.

6   Torrance GW, Furlong W, Feeny D, Boyle M. Multi-attribute preference functions. Health utilities index. *Pharmacoeconomics* 1995;**7**:503–20.

7   Euroqol Group. Euroqol – a new facility for the measurement of health-related quality of life. *Health Policy* 1990;**16**:199–208.

8   MVH Group. *The Measurement and Valuation of Health: First Report on the Main Survey*. York: Centre for Health Economics, University of York, 1994.

9   Johnson J, Coons SJ, Ergo A, Szava-Kovats G. Valuation of EuroQOL (EQ-5D) health states in an adult US sample. *Pharmacoeconomics* 1998;**13**:421–33.

10 Gafni A, Birch S. Searching for a common currency: critical appraisal of the scientific basis underlying European harmonization of the measurement of Health Related Quality of Life (Euroqol). *Health Policy* 1993;**23**:219–28

11 Brazier J, Deverill M, Green C, Harper R, Booth A. A review of the use of health status measures in economic evaluation. *Health Technol Assess* 1999;**3**(9).

12 Froberg DG, Kane RL. Methodology for measuring health-state preferences– II scaling methods. *J Clin Epidemiol* 1989;**42**:459–71.

13 Torrance GW. Measurement of health state utilities for economic appraisal: a review. *J Health Economics* 1986;**5**:1–30.

14 Johnston K, Brown J, Gerard K, O'Hanlon M, Morton A. Valuing temporary and chronic health states associated with breast screening. *Soc Sci Med* 1998;**47**:213–22.

15 Torrance GW, Thomas WH, Sackett DL. A utility maximization model for evaluation of health care programmes. *Health Serv Res* 1972;**7**:118–33.

16 Mehrez A, Gafni A. Quality adjusted life years, utility theory, and healthy years equivalents. *Med Decis Making* 1989;**9**:142–9.

17 Culyer AJ, Wagstaff A. QALYs and HYEs. *J Health Economics* 1993;**11**:311–23.

18 Loomes G. The myth of the HYE. *J Health Economics* 1995;**14**:1–8.

19 Gafni A, Birch S, Mehrez A. Economics, health and health economics: HYEs versus QALYs. *J Health Economics* 1993;**11**:325–39.

20 Mehrez A, Gafni A. Healthy years equivalents versus quality adjusted life years: in pursuit of progress. *Med Decis Making* 1993;**13**:287–92.

21 Donaldson C, Shackley P. Does "process utility" exist? A case study of willingness to pay for laparoscopic cholecystectomy. *Soc Sci Med* 1997;**44**:699–707.

22 Johannesson M, Jonsson B. Economic evaluation in health care: is there a role for cost-benefit analysis? *Health Policy* 1991;**17**:1–23.

23 Shackley P, Ryan M. Involving consumers in health care decision making. *Health Care Analysis* 1995;**3**:196–204.

24 Ryan M. *Using Conjoint Analysis in Health Care to Elicit Patients' Preferences*. London: Office of Health Economics, 1996.

25 Diamond P, J Hausman. Contingent valuation: is some number better than no number? *J Econ Perspectives* 1994;**8**:45–64.

26 Olsen JA, Donaldson C. Helicopters, hearts and hips: using willingness to pay to set priorities for public sector health care programmes. *Soc Sci Med* 1998;**46**:1–12.

27 Donaldson C. *Developing the Method of "Willingness to Pay" for Assessment of Community Preferences for Health Care*. Final report to Biomed 2

Programme (PL950832) of the European Commission. Health Economics Research Unit, University of Aberdeen and Departments of Economics and Community Health Sciences, University of Calgary, 1999.

28   O'Shea E, Stewart J, Donaldson C. Eliciting preferences for resource allocation for health care. *Econ Soc Rev* 2002;**32**:217–38.

29   Shackley P, Donaldson C. Using willingness to pay to elicit community preferences for health care: is an incremental approach the way forward? *J Health Economics* 2002;**21**:971–91.

30   Stewart J, O'Shea E, Donaldson C, Shackley P. Do ordering effects matter in willingness to pay studies of health care? *J Health Economics* 2002;**21**:585–99.

31   Donaldson C, Hundley V, Mapp T. Willingness to pay: a method for measuring preferences for maternity care? *Birth* 1998;**25**:33–40.

32   Farrar S, Ryan M, Ross D, Ludbrook A. Using discrete choice modelling in priority setting: an application to clinical service developments. *Soc Sci Med* 2000;**50**:63–75.

11: The challenge of involving the public

Introduction

A further important issue, yet to be addressed directly in the Toolkit, is the involvement of the public in priority setting. After over three decades of debate, it is becoming more and more accepted that the public should have some role to play in priority setting in health care. The primary focus of this chapter is on involving the public through eliciting principles and developing criteria on which decision makers base funding decisions. At the end of the chapter, the notion of eliciting preferences for health care and health states is again touched on, as the methods of discrete choice experiments (DCEs) and willingness to pay (WTP), described in Chapter 10, are an important part of the potential contribution of economics to public involvement. Although a comprehensive assessment is not provided, references will enable the reader to explore issues in greater depth.

Rationale for using the public

A number of reasons in favour of public consultation in priority setting have been advanced in the literature including the following[1-3]:

- a desire, particularly in primarily publicly funded health care contexts, to share ownership in rationing decisions
- to make providers more accountable to the public
- an acceptance that public engagement is central to democratic theory
- a realisation that citizens bring different types of knowledge to decision making processes.

That said, it should also be recognised that involving the public in healthcare priority setting comes with a number of issues requiring careful consideration. One such issue is that the public (as well as healthcare professionals) may receive a skewed set of information when it comes to identifying priorities in health care. Coverage in the media often focuses on "bricks and mortar" and the latest high technology pieces of equipment, with less attention given to health promotion and prevention strategies. Thus, if the public is to be engaged, biases brought to the table must be carefully assessed, just as should be the case with consultation from any stakeholder. Further, education on healthcare organisation, social determinants of health, ethical principles and health economic concepts may be required prior to obtaining informed input from members of the public.

Another important issue is that in any public consultation, those with a keen interest, and those already empowered in society, are more likely to become engaged.[4] In fact, broad representation may not readily be achieved in many cases, as input can become isolated to special interests or personal experiences, potentially resulting in the health of the population as a whole not being well served by the input of a relatively small number.

The intention here is not to enter into a lengthy debate about these issues, but rather to raise points which require careful consideration when decisions are being made about engaging the public in priority setting. A starting place for moving forward is the recognition that public consultation is an important input to the priority setting process, but must be balanced with other sources of evidence and the input of other stakeholders. As Wiseman *et al.* state "priority setting should be informed by the preferences of more than one group".[3] Still, the question remains, if public input is to be sought, what exactly should be elicited for the purposes of setting priorities?

Information to gain from the public

Returning to the literature, a convergence of viewpoints has arisen, whereby both decision makers and the public seem to be in favour of public involvement in the form of developing key objectives, or principles, on which decision makers can then make funding decisions. For example, a recent study in

Britain found that members of the public favoured an "accountable consultation" role for system and programme level decisions, but a reluctance to have input into specific treatment decisions.[2] A study in Sydney, Australia, based on a large convenience sample of citizens, also found that the public wants input particularly in prioritisation processes across broad service areas, including development of the criteria on which funding decisions will ultimately be based.[3] Similarly, decision makers involved in work in Alberta have suggested that a means of operationalising public involvement would be to engage the public in developing criteria for the decision makers to then use in priority setting activity. Using public input in this manner would also appear to be supported in other studies,[1] and fits with the notion of a healthcare constitution, advanced by Mooney.[5]

Of course, it may be that in some organisations, the public will not want to be involved in priority setting in any fashion, and thus this should be investigated locally prior to efforts being made to elicit public input regarding principles or criteria.[6] As well, the "public" can take different forms, and ultimately a value judgement is required to determine who should and should not be involved and even who should be making that decision! As alluded to above, empirical work would support a more pluralistic approach to citizenry involvement which can include both interested citizens and random samples of citizens.[7] In the end, the expected role of the public should be made explicit,[1] and clear rationale should be put forth detailing why input from certain groups was elicited.

Methods for engaging the public

If the public does want to be involved, and decision makers are receptive to receiving input for priority setting from the local citizenry, numerous methods are available. Broadly speaking, citizens can be directly involved in the priority setting process or can be engaged through various qualitative and quantitative approaches in order to obtain information which is then used by decision makers. A recent example of direct public participation comes from a study in Ontario, Canada, where a small number of citizens, acting as either public or patient representatives, worked alongside clinical and managerial decision makers in determining priorities in cancer and cardiac care.[8] It was reported that these members of the public had little or no contribution to technical discussions such as the effectiveness and cost-effectiveness of specific treatments, but were able to provide useful perspectives about values and criteria.

Of course, the challenge in engaging the public in this way is that only a very small number of individuals can participate. To address this, the advisory panel in a programme budgeting and marginal analysis (PBMA) exercise in Scotland set up and advertised a community phone line to elicit suggestions for options for change within the health organisation.[9] However, they reported a relatively small number of calls to the line, and further it might be suggested that only individuals with a vested interest in a particular programme would call in. The other point to make, though, is that depending on the scope of the priority setting exercise, representation of the entire citizenry may not be the primary objective, and in some cases vested parties may provide valuable information.

A number of authors have presented various methods for eliciting public input when the public does not have a seat directly at the decision making table.[1,4,10] Several such methods are outlined in Table 11.1. Choice of which method to use depends on the context and specific objective for eliciting public views, as well as the time-line and availability of resources. A recent, extensive review of this literature concluded that there is no gold standard for involving the public, and further, that a combination of methods is likely preferred.[11]

In applying one or more of these methods, various techniques can be employed. For example, participants can be presented with a series of criteria in a questionnaire format and then be asked to rank them or to provide relative weightings. As well, more than one of the above methods can be utilised. For example, a focus group could be used to generate a list of principles, then, building on this, a quantitative survey could be used to elicit the weights for these criteria. Further, the public does not have to be asked directly about relevant principles to get insight into those principles. If ascertaining the relative value of extension of life

Table 11.1 Methods for eliciting public input in priority setting

Method	Description and comments
Quantitative surveys	• Responses to standardised questions are elicited, either as telephone or postal questionnaires, or face to face interviews • Sampling can be done through using telephone books or electoral rolls, and can be random or non-random in nature • As the sampling frame is often incomplete, marginalised groups may not be well represented
Qualitative interviews	• Non-standardised, indepth interviews to identify perceptions and experiences of respondents • Random or purposive sampling can be used, noting that the purpose is usually not to obtain generalisable results but rather deeper insight into specific issues
Public meetings	• Can be held at national, regional or local level, through which key issues can be discussed and community preferences elicited • Exhibited preferences at such meetings are likely to differ significantly from those of the general public due to the special interest groups such forums attract
Focus groups	• Small group meeting in which some aspect of public perceptions are assessed • Difficult to get representation of the general public, although as with qualitative surveys, this may not be the intention
Citizen juries	• Representative panel of citizens meet over several days to hear evidence on a particular issue and then deliver a "verdict" • Not particularly relevant if the objective is to obtain principles or criteria for the public, as it is more geared as a decision making process
Advisory panels	• Representative citizens (or patients) are selected and brought together routinely to discuss issues and provide opinions • Can improve the visibility and accountability of decision making processes and provide relevant insight for decision makers

versus quality of life is thought to be important, choices about the balance of healthcare dollars spent for life saving services versus services that improve quality of life could be discussed, for example, at a public meeting.

Eliciting community preferences

The focus to this point has been on involving the public as "accountable consultants" for the primary purpose of obtaining criteria or principles which in turn would serve as the basis for rationing decisions. Another important way in which the public can be involved is in eliciting community preferences for health care or health states. Economic techniques like WTP and DCEs can be used for this purpose. As described in Chapter 10, the idea would be to obtain preferences for a specific service or health state, and then feed such information directly into the priority setting process in a health organisation.

For example, referring back to the Norwegian WTP study on hearts, hips and helicopters in Chapter 10, the values elicited from members of the public could be directly incorporated into a marginal analysis advisory panel charged with setting priorities and allocating resources. Similarly, a DCE could be conducted to elicit patient preferences for a particular service. Such information could then be passed on to a decision making group responsible for deciding how best to spend the limited resources allocated to the given programme.

To date, there have been limited examples of using economic techniques like WTP and DCE to directly support priority setting activity in the manner discussed here. However, as the validity of the methods improve, and an understanding of these techniques by decision makers is gained, one might expect to see this type of quantification of public preferences in routine use by decision makers in priority setting processes in the near future.

Summary

In summary, it would seem that the public does want to be involved in priority setting in health care, although confirmation of this should be sought in local contexts. The literature would support the use of public input for developing the principles or criteria on which decision makers can then base specific funding decisions. There are various means of eliciting such information, and in the end, the specific approach taken will depend on the scope of the priority setting exercise in question and the type of information sought, as well as the time and resources available. As well, as discussed in detail in Chapter 10 and reviewed in brief here, the public can also be used to elicit preferences for health care or health states using techniques like WTP and DCEs. The key is to be explicit about what is being sought and the means by which this is to be done.

References

1 Lomas J. Reluctant rationers: public input to health care priorities. *J Health Serv Res Policy* 1997;2:103–111.
2 Litva A, Coast J, Donovan J *et al.* "The public is too subjective": public involvement at different levels of health-care decision making. *Soc Sci Med* 2002;54:1825–37.
3 Wiseman V, Mooney G, Berry G, Tang KC. Involving the general public in priority setting: experiences from Australia. *Soc Sci Med* 2003;56:1001–12.
4 Donovan J, Coast J. Public participation in priority setting: commitment or illusion? In: Cost J, Donovan J, Frankel S eds. *Priority Setting: the Health Care Debate.* London: John Wiley & Sons Ltd, 1996.
5 Mooney G. "Communitarian claims" as an ethical basis for allocating health care resources. *Soc Sci Med* 1998;47:1171–80.
6 Mooney G, Gerard K. QALY league tables: handle with care. *Health Economics* 1993;2:59–64.
7 Abelson J, Lomas J, Eyles J, Birch S, Veenstra G. Does the community want devolved authority? Results of deliberative polling in Ontario. *Can Med Assoc J* 1995;153:403–12
8 Martin D, Abelson J, Singer P. Participation in health care priority-setting through the eyes of the participants. *J Health Serv Res Policy* 2002;7:222–9.
9 Ruta D, Donaldson C, Gilray I. Economics, public health and health care purchasing: the Tayside experience of programme budgeting and marginal analysis. *J Health Serv Res Policy* 1996;1:185–93.
10 Mullen P. Public involvement in health care priority setting: an overview of methods for eliciting values. *Health Expectations* 1999;2:222–34.
11 Menon D, Stafinski T, Martin D, Windwick B, Singer P, Caulfield T. *Incorporating Public Values and Technical Information in to Health Care Resource Allocation Decision-making.* Edmonton: Alberta Heritage Foundation for Medical Research, 2003.

12: The challenge of the organisation

Introduction

The final challenge has to do not so much with economics *per se*, or a given methodology for setting priorities in health organisations, but rather with the nature and culture of the organisation itself. One of the major challenges to the implementation of an explicit, evidence-based approach to priority setting in health care is that of organisational behaviour. Some of the important questions in relation to the context in which priority setting occurs include the following:

- Can a culture of openness to change be fostered, in order that health organisations move away from offering entrenched services in favour of a process of informed assessment and delivery of new models of care based on evidence and local expert opinion?
- What are some of the organisational and managerial barriers and facilitators to using an explicit approach to priority setting?
- How can an approach to priority setting be integrated into core business and strategic planning so that priority setting is not confined to one-off exercises in isolated parts of the organisation?
- What kind of incentive systems might assist decision makers in moving towards informed, explicit priority setting activity?
- How are physicians to be engaged in priority setting so as to foster both accountability and buy-in for the policy decisions being made?

To aid in addressing these issues, relevant insight from priority setting work carried out in Australia and Canada is discussed, and a review of the relevant management and institutionalist economics literatures is provided. First, though, this challenge of the organisation is laid out in more detail.

The challenge of the organisation

Several years ago, a survey of decision makers was conducted in two UK health organisations, the Newcastle Health Authority and the Grampian Health Board.[1,2] The surveys found that there was dissatisfaction with historical allocation processes, and that a mapping of priorities through the use of programme budgeting would be seen as very helpful. Further, managers, for the most part, wanted a system that would provide greater accountability of public funds. However, those surveyed did not feel that further organisational change, in the form of introducing an explicit approach to priority setting, would be beneficial due to the many changes that had already taken place in the National Health Service (NHS) over the previous number of years. As well, they articulated that any new tool should be consistent with the existing health strategy. The points raised through these surveys suggest that although an approach like programme budgeting and marginal analysis (PBMA) may be viewed favourably, organisationally speaking, there could be resistance in implementation. These studies also suggested that more work would be required on how explicit approaches to priority setting are best incorporated into routine decision making processes within health organisations.

This discussion can be extended beyond the use of priority setting frameworks, to include the uptake of specific results from tools like economic evaluations,[3] and more broadly, the uptake of evidence to inform decision making processes.[4] For the reader of this book, it is hoped that there is some leaning towards implementing explicit priority setting strategies in one's own organisation. However, there is also a necessary recognition that willingness of this kind may be met with resistance that is outside the control of the individual decision maker.

Addressing the challenge

Australian insight

In the late 1990s, Peacock[5] put forth a number of issues, based on empirical observation, for consideration in the development and application of PBMA as a practical decision making aid. These include:

- the need for relative organisational stability in the given health organisation
- a degree of integration in funding and priority setting mechanisms
- acceptance by stakeholders of needing to examine both costs and benefits in decision making
- presence of strong organisational leadership and change management strategies
- involvement of clinicians from the outset of the priority setting process
- provision of education by researchers on key economic concepts and priority setting processes
- a commitment by the health organisation to ongoing refinement of approaches to priority setting.

In addition, based on this work in Australia, it was found that a successful application of PBMA will likely rest on:

- the initial programme of choice
- availability of information systems and cost data
- how the lists for expansion and reduction are generated
- whether specific decision analysis techniques like option appraisal are used to estimate benefits in the marginal analysis.

If the primary challenges of PBMA lie more with a fit with the organisational context rather than the approach itself, the information challenges posed by Peacock become critical in understanding the uptake and ultimate longer term use of the "economic way of thinking" in health organisations.

Canadian insight

Building on this work in Australia, we embarked on a project in Alberta, Canada which in part had as its aim to identify specific barriers and facilitators to informed, explicit priority setting activity in health organisations.[6] Out of this work, a model of the PBMA process was depicted, as seen in

Figure 6.3. This model draws out some of the important organisational barriers and facilitators to the uptake of PBMA and ultimate follow-through of recommendations. It also highlights issues for the development and application of PBMA as a practical decision making aid, and serves as a summary of important issues identified in this Alberta-based research project.

In essence, the model stresses the need to consider priority setting activity within the context in which it is to be carried out. Noting the points raised from Peacock's work in Australia, and the model for priority setting from Alberta, decision makers can begin to gauge whether the environment is right for embarking on a priority setting process which is both explicit and informed. Of course, it may well be that parts of a given organisation are more ready then other areas, and thus the introduction of a PBMA-like approach can occur in one programme area even if significant barriers exist in other programme areas. Table 12.1 outlines the key organisational issues requiring consideration, at the outset of and during application of an explicit approach to priority setting, as identified through the recent work in Australia and Canada.

Management literature

In order to more fully develop the issues presented above, insight can also be drawn from the broader healthcare management and organisational behaviour literature. At a group or individual level, Shortell and Kaluzny argue that change is best understood as a process,[6] and, like others,[7-9] puts forth a multi-staged description of this process. The basic steps include:

- awareness that there is a gap between what is being done and what should be done
- identification of key discrepancies
- operationalising the change
- institutionalising the change into ongoing activities.

In some ways, these steps provide a theoretical backdrop with which the model outlined in Figure 6.3 can be compared.

Table 12.1 Organisational issues requiring consideration

Considerations when embarking on explicit priority setting	Considerations as the priority setting process gets going	Considerations nearing the end of the priority setting process
Relative organisational stability	Examination of both costs and benefits in relation to a set of pre-defined, locally generated criteria	Commitment to ongoing refinement/iteration of priority setting process
Strong leadership and change management strategies	Education on economic concepts	Resources earmarked for making recommended changes
Integration of budgets to allow for reallocation of resources	Integration of priority setting approach with budget processes	Continued fostering of trust between stakeholders
Culture to learn and openness to change	Participation of clinicians	Decision makers have authority to ensure changes followed through
Resources earmarked for priority setting process	Approach consistent with existing managerial activity	Incentive system developed to engage all relevant stakeholders

Research on decision makers using economic evaluations in practice has highlighted two major types of barriers, namely those related to "accessibility" and those related to "acceptability".[*,10,11] Barriers of accessibility relate to difficulties in accessing pertinent information and the lack of relevant interpretation skills, while issues of acceptability relate to the supply of information in a timely fashion and the quality of the information as it pertains to a given decision making context. For example, it has been suggested that economic evaluation results are often ignored because of the inability to shift resources across budgets in the health sector.[11] In

*The authors acknowledge Professor Stirling Bryan, University of Birmingham, UK, for drawing this line of work to their attention.

Table 12.2 Barriers and facilitators to change in organisations

Barriers	Facilitators
Lack of vision	Effective leadership
Discontinuity of staff	Commitment to vision
Lack of resources	Changing incentives
Inadequate training	Individual knowledge, skills and attitudes
Negative previous experience with change	Preparedness for change
Inability to shift resources across budgets	Resource availability

addition, Jick[12] reports that the supporting structures or mechanisms in the organisation will influence change, as well as whether there is a vision from senior management that has been directed to the operational managers and the political dynamics of the change.

Based on work from the management literature,[11,13–17] several barriers and facilitators to change are summarised in Table 12.2. As different contexts will require different strategies, it is best to have a process in place for identification of barriers, and plans to overcome those barriers, prior to embarking on a priority setting process. As well, an understanding of the "antecedent conditions" in the organisation can be used to strategically plan whether the time and setting are most receptive to explicit priority setting activity. Finally, there also must be one person with change responsibility, and there needs to be an environment where learning and innovation are held as key values.

Institutional economics literature

Another lens through which to examine priority setting, as it relates to the organisation, comes from the institutional economics literature. An institutionalist approach holds that economic development does not occur in isolation from institutional or structural factors in society.[18] The argument here is that as conventionally understood, economic evaluation does not serve to capture all relevant factors in its analysis. Factors such as community values, infrastructure support and social capital all play a role in affecting health, in addition to the specific healthcare services provided to individuals. Thus, in analysing how best to spend the limited resources available, one should take on a more "holistic" view, in part through recognising the organisational and structural influences affecting the health of individuals in the population.

This same literature can also be tapped into to look at the role of incentives in priority setting activity. It has been argued that the success of a PBMA exercise relies on the goodwill of the participants in providing a realistic assessment of expected benefits.[19] It can be observed, however, that decision makers have an incentive to overestimate expected benefits for their proposed growth items and underestimate expected benefits lost for their own disinvestment proposals. As there is status attached to the biggest budget, there is an incentive for managers to want to attract funding for their growth options, and also to prevent funding to be taken from their areas. The problem is that this incentive may be at odds with what is the most efficient use of resources from the perspective of the organisation as a whole.

The argument continues that the potential gaming associated with a PBMA exercise can result in transaction costs, such as the need to validate the claims of other managers involved in the priority setting activity.[19] Thus, the incentive for each manager to participate equates to the potential gain in terms of an increase in their budget resulting from the PBMA activity less any ensuing transaction costs. Of course, most methods of allocation incur some transaction costs, such as those related to lobbying or politicising a particular issue. In any case, the transaction cost issue is one that is not generally considered in the assessment of priority setting approaches, and could have important implications as to whether using an approach like PBMA is "efficient" in and of itself.

Several solutions have been presented to alleviate transaction costs associated with the organisational incentives faced by decision makers.[19] These include increasing the information base for assessing costs and benefits of resources shifts and making such information available to all participants in the exercise, as well as utilising external, non-vested parties to monitor the validity of the proposals. These institutional responses, however, are likely to have associated administrative costs, which must be balanced against the transaction costs they are trying to minimise. In the end, it is useful to think through the incentives to participate in explicit priority setting activity, noting that unexpected costs to the organisation may result.

Coupling this institutionalist economics insight with the broader organisational considerations raised above, through empirical observation and review of the literature, begins to identify the many related issues that need addressing at the outset of, or during, the priority setting process.

Related issues: incentives and physicians

Two issues of relevance to this discussion of using an explicit approach to priority setting in the real world of health organisations are:

- having a set of incentives to encourage participation in priority setting activity and to reward efficient behaviour
- engaging physicians in the processes at hand.

Aspects of the first issue have already been addressed in the previous subsection on institutional economics, while the second involves issues which, if fully articulated, would fall well beyond the scope of this Toolkit. Nonetheless, in order to illustrate several specific points these two issues are now addressed directly.

Incentives in priority setting

The need for incentives

It is a fact that everyone responds to incentives.[20] Physicians are not "bad" because they may, in some instances, drive excess demand due to their salary being based on fee for service. Similarly, managers are not "bad" for wanting to take action to stay within budget in order to receive an annual bonus. In both these examples, people are merely responding to the incentives before them. The key is thus in providing the right incentives to foster behaviour that is in line with the aims and objectives of a given health organisation or healthcare system. Here, incentives as they pertain to engaging stakeholders in priority setting activity are first examined, before touching on the use of incentives to reward efficient and innovative behaviour. Following this, an example is briefly outlined of incentives being misaligned.

Engaging stakeholders

Engagement in an explicit approach to priority setting can be fostered through providing both "structural" incentives and "programme" incentives. A major reason for not participating in a process which, as part of the activity involves identifying areas for improving efficiency and proposing disinvestments, is that most healthcare budgets, as was discussed in Chapter 3, are based on what was spent in the previous year. That is, if a programme area or health organisation offers services using less resources than was budgeted, the tendency has been to reduce the following year's budget by the amount left over. This creates a clear disincentive for coming in under budget.

What is required is a positive feedback loop which would see structural incentives that foster behaviour in line with identifying areas to release resources for reallocation to growth areas so that overall benefit can be improved, or other important criteria can be met. One way to do this is to have more sophisticated monitoring of expenditure, so the reward or penalty is not based simply on what was spent, but rather on whether the spend was appropriate. While this may be difficult to implement in lieu of formal evidence to rate resource allocation decisions, it is this way of thinking which would be of value when moving towards a more explicit approach for priority setting.

In relation, a programme incentive might include gain sharing of some form. That is, if an individual programme area is required to come up with efficiency improvements, all resources that are released in that area do not necessarily have to go to the central pool for reinvestment elsewhere. A percentage of the resources released from efficiency improvements could stay within that programme area for reinvestment in existing or newly proposed services. Of course, some managers may be sceptical of the incentive system and suggest that they will keep all of their budget if they do identify any opportunities for improving efficiency. Thus, this type of programme incentive should be invoked in conjunction with changing the reward/penalty system of coming in under budget.

Rewarding innovative and efficient behaviour

In addition to engaging players in explicit priority setting processes, another aspect of incentives is to directly reward innovative and efficient behaviour. An innovative behaviour could be described as taking a longer term view of health and investing in a health promoting activity, or taking a measurable investment risk when the evidence on the suspected return is even more uncertain than normal. A key disincentive to innovative behaviour is if personnel believe that the organisation will not make a credible commitment to recommended options for change.[20] Thus, organisationally, there must be a demonstrated collective will that not only will health promotion, for example, be supported on paper, but that strategic investment with actual dollars will follow. Then, decision makers will sense that it is acceptable to invest upstream in a health promoting activity vis-à-vis an explicit choice not to invest downstream in acute care.

In terms of efficient behaviour, any number of non-financial incentives can serve as rewards, including reduced waiting times for patients, enhancements to ambulatory care services, and better equipment. Another positive incentive for encouraging efficient behaviour is greater access to professional development opportunities. Continuing education enhances staff skills and exposes them to other models through meetings with their peers. These learning opportunities, in turn, may promote innovative ideas in the organisation. Of course, direct financial incentives can be evoked as well,[21] although this may provide still other incentives which may counter the initial intended effect.

Misalignment of incentives

One final issue with respect to incentives is in relation to the respective roles of physicians and health organisations in some contexts. The issue is that when physicians are paid on a fee for service basis, they have an incentive to drive service utilisation. Conversely, where health organisations hold fiscal accountability to the ministry and public, they have an incentive to constrain costs. The problem arises, in particular, in contexts where physicians and health organisations have no formal relationship. For example, if the physicians are not directly accountable to a health organisation, the organisation cannot tightly control the services provided. Thus, while the health organisation may be compelled to limit patient access to certain services, physicians, who are not employees of the organisation, may resist having their treatment decisions dictated by administrators, especially if they feel that they are offering best practices.

What this all amounts to is that physicians do not have an incentive to improve efficiency overall if it will result in funding, equipment or human resource reductions in their service area. The mismatched incentives between physicians and health organisations translate into a lack of constancy of purpose, poor cooperation and contradictory targets. What is required to rectify this situation is either movement away from fee for service reimbursement mechanisms, or development, if not already in place, of more formal relationships between physicians and health organisations, whereby physicians could hold more fiscal accountability for their utilisation decisions. This issue, as mentioned, is beyond the scope of the Toolkit, but is presented here to illustrate that even with other incentive-related changes, challenges to changing practice in certain contexts will still exist unless the issue of the relationship between physicians and health organisations is addressed.

Incentives summary

In summary, an explicit approach to priority setting should include incentives to engage stakeholders and stimulate innovative and efficient behaviour. Changes in how budgets are set, and inclusion of gain sharing propositions, can aid in fostering stakeholder participation. Credible organisational commitment and incentives in the form of funding for personnel, equipment or professional development can be applied to reward innovation and improved efficiency. Finally, aligning incentives between physicians and the health organisations is an important issue requiring attention in some contexts, and may help to explain slow uptake of recommendations through priority setting, even when other incentive systems have been put in place.

Physician involvement in priority setting

Importance of physician involvement

The need for physician involvement in the organisations with which they work is becoming increasingly recognised.[22-24] However, most of the research on this issue to date has focused on physician involvement in healthcare governance[25] or change management processes more broadly[26] as opposed to direct participation in priority setting. Due to the role physicians play in most health systems, at least some involvement in policy making practices should be favoured. Further, physicians, like other clinical staff, have a wealth of information that would go untapped without involvement in some form.

Challenges to physician involvement

While physician engagement in priority setting is likely to be supported in principle by the various stakeholders, there are numerous challenges in engaging physicians in priority setting activity. One problem is that physicians may claim to not have the time to participate in activities which they might view as "administratively driven". Another key issue is that as direct service providers, physicians face different pressures than administrators. As such, they often feel less able to reduce or cut services, making priority setting difficult, particularly at a broad level across different services. While health organisation decision makers are generally removed from individual patients who are demanding services, physicians feel primary responsibility to their patients, sometimes placing them at odds with notions such as disinvestment.

Roles for physicians

Despite these challenges, physicians are likely to have the most influence on implementing operational change within health organisations.[26] Thus, what role might physicians play specifically in priority setting activity? One option is that as physicians have more intimate knowledge of the pressures in their specific areas, they can thus serve as a valuable resource in supporting activity involving resource reallocation. That is, the "expert opinion" of physicians in specific areas should be drawn out and fed into priority setting activity. Another role is to provide the evidence to support service delivery, and to lead in innovations and new approaches that may save resources and/or improve health outcomes. As it is often the practitioners who know the literature in the specific clinical areas in the most detail, drawing on physicians and other clinicians to provide evidence from research and other sources can be critical to making the best decisions locally. In addition, physicians can provide a "validity-check" function, whereby once initial investment and disinvestment options are developed by a given advisory panel, various stakeholder groups, including physicians, can review the options and provide additional input prior to final recommendations being made.

Still another option would be to have physicians sit as members of advisory panels charged with weighing options for investment and disinvestment. While this may well be appropriate within specific service areas, caution should be exerted in including individual physicians on an advisory panel which has as its aim to reallocate resources broadly across service areas. The rationale, as alluded to above, is that physicians may find themselves in a conflict of interest, wanting to be advocates for their patients yet needing to take a broader system view in macro-oriented priority setting. Thus, unless physicians hold a non-clinical administrative post and are expected as part of that job to partake directly in priority setting activity across broad service areas, using physicians to support priority setting at a broad level, through providing evidence and expert advice, may be the best road to take.

Physician involvement summary

In summary, as innovations in clinical practice are often driven by physicians and other clinical leaders, input from the clinicians should be actively incorporated into priority setting. The role physicians are to play will undoubtedly vary depending on the context and prior level of engagement in priority setting processes, but physicians should, at a minimum, have input in discussion on best practice. This will provide insight into the clinical realities of service delivery and as well may bring evidence forward to inform reallocation decisions. In priority setting at a programmatic level, such input could take place through having physicians sit directly on an advisory panel. For broader processes, input from physicians should be sought, but recommendations for reallocation should in most cases be driven primarily by those who have a wider mandate.

Conclusion

There are no easy solutions to the challenge of the organisation as it pertains to the use of an explicit approach to priority setting. Indeed, this challenge alone may go a long way in explaining why various approaches to aid decision makers in weighing up treatment options and setting priorities often have limited use in practice. Thinking through barriers and facilitators to explicit, evidence-based priority setting activity, at the outset, will likely save time and resources in the long run. In short, context matters. There is nothing about PBMA *per se*, other than its adaptability, that will ensure success. Fostering the right environment is crucial. Specific suggestions for moving forward within a given organisational context were provided in this chapter and can be drawn upon accordingly. Finally, time spent developing a locally targeted incentive system and endeavouring to engage physicians in priority setting should prove fruitful over time.

Importantly, all of the issues discussed in this chapter fall beyond the scope of any one discipline. Expertise from health economists, managers, clinicians and organisational behaviourists is required to move these discussions forward.

References

1 Miller P. Managing informed purchasing: a survey of decision makers. *J Manage Med* 1997;**11**:35–42.
2 Vale L. *Programme Budgeting: Key Decision Makers Survey.* Aberdeen: Grampian Health Board, 1996.
3 Ross J. The use of economic evaluation in health care: Australian decision makers' perceptions. *Health Policy* 1995;**31**:103–10.
4 Ferlie E, Fitzgerald L, Wood M. Getting evidence into clinical practice: an organisational behaviour perspective. *J Health Serv Res Policy* 2000;**5**: 96–102.
5 Peacock S. *An Evaluation of Program Budgeting and Marginal Analysis Applied in South Australian Hospitals.* Melbourne: Centre for Health Program Evaluation, Monash University, 1998.
6 Shortell S, Kaluzny A, eds. *Health Care Management: Organisation Design and Behaviour.* New York: Delmar Publishers Inc, 1994.
7 Rogers EM. *Diffusion of Innovations, 4th edn.* New York: The Free Press, 1995.
8 Spasoff RA. *Epidemiologic Methods for Health Policy.* New York: Oxford University Press, 1999.
9 Mink OG, Esterhuysen PW, Mink BP, Owen KQ. *Change at Work: A Comprehensive Management Process for Transforming Organisations.* San Francisco: Jossey-Bass Publishers, 1993.
10 Kernick DP. The impact of health economics on healthcare delivery. *Pharmacoeconomics* 2000;**18**:311–15.
11 Von der Schulenburg J, ed. *The influence of economic evaluation studies on health care decision-making.* Amsterdam: IOS Press, 2001.
12 Jick TD. *Managing Change: cases and concepts.* Boston: Richard D. Irwin Inc., 1993.
13 Daley JM, Kettner PM. The episode of purposive change. *J Community Dev Soc* 1986;**17**:54–72.
14 Lorenzi NM, Riley RT. Managing change: an overview. *J Am Med Informatics Assoc* 2000;**7**:116–24.
15 Grol R, Grimshaw J. Evidence-based implementation of evidence-based medicine. *J Quality Improvement* 1999;**25**:503–13.
16 Beckhard R, Harris RT. *Organisational Transitions, 2nd edn.* Reading, Mass: Addison-Wesley Publishing Company, Inc, 1987.
17 Ash JS, Anderson JG, Gorman PN *et al.* Managing change: analysis of a hypothetical case. *J Am Med Informatics Assoc* 2000;**7**:125–34.
18 Jan S. A holistic approach to the economic evaluation of health programs using institutionalist methodology. *Soc Sci Med* 1998;**47**:1565–72.
19 Jan. S. Institutional considerations in priority setting: transactions cost perspective on PBMA. *Health Economics* 2000;**9**:631–41.
20 Jan S. A perspective on the analysis of credible commitment and myopia in health sector decision making. *Health Policy* 2002;**53**:269–78.

21 Bailit Health Purchasing. *Provider Incentive Models for Improving Quality of Care*. Washington, DC: Academy for Health Services Research and Health Policy, 2002.
22 Burns LR, Walston SL, Alexander JA *et al*. Just how integrated are integrated delivery systems? Results from a national survey. *Health Care Manage Rev* 2001;**26**:20–39.
23 The Accreditation Council for Graduate Medical Education *GME Core Curriculum*. Chicago: ACGME, 2000
24 The Royal College of Physicians and Surgeons of Canada. *Skills for the New Millennium: Report of the Societal Needs Working Group Can MEDS 2000 Project*. Ottawa: RCPSC, 1996.
25 Kocher C, Kumar K, Subramaniam R. Physician-hospital integration strategies: impact on physicians involvement in hospital governance. *Health Care Manage Rev* 1998;**23**:38–47.
26 Silversin J, Kornacki MJ. *Leading Physicians Through Change*. Tampa, Florida: American College of Physician Executives, 2000.

Part 5: Conclusions

13: Toolkit summary and recommendations

Concepts and tools

The starting point for setting priorities in health care is the recognition that resources are scarce. That is, there are not enough resources to fund all the claims on those resources. The implication of this is that choices need to be made between what to fund and what not to fund. As health economics is the study of choice, it is plausible that an approach to priority setting based on an economic way of thinking could serve as a reasonable base for moving forward. The approach for priority setting put forth here, to operationalise this economic way of thinking, is programme budgeting and marginal analysis, or PBMA.

The economics behind PBMA, covered in the first half of the Toolkit, are actually fairly simple. The initial concept is that of opportunity cost, which carries with it the understanding that in investing resources in one spot, some opportunity for benefit, through investing those resources elsewhere, has been lost. The key in setting priorities, then, is to measure or weigh out the costs and benefits of doing one thing vis-à-vis another. The other concept is that of the margin, which is about shifting or changing the resource mix. If the budget increases, one could reasonably ask how best the additional resources should be spent. Conversely, if the budget decreases, one would likely want to take resources from areas which are producing the least benefit. If the budget was neither increasing nor decreasing, the question remains as to whether resources should be reallocated so as to improve benefit to the population being served. In theory, the process of shifting resources across major service areas, or across programmes within service areas, should be conducted until the marginal cost to marginal benefit ratios of each of the services or programmes is equal. In practice, such shifting is likely fundamental to the long term survival and ultimate sustainability of one's health organisation.

Of course, there are many approaches for setting priorities in health care, including the most common method, that being allocation based on historical patterns. Assuming the intention is to get the most out of the available resources, approaches for setting priorities should be considered in light of the economic concepts of opportunity cost and the margin. Approaches which are not based on these economic concepts include needs assessment and defining core services. Needs assessment is problematic as the focus is on the size of the problem or gaps in services as opposed to the benefit that can be obtained from services or interventions.[1] As well, this approach generally does not consider the impact on resources. Defining core services is problematic as if a service is "out", but more benefit at the margin would be derived by investing there vis-à-vis cutting back on some service that is "in", shifting of resources from the "in" service to the "out" service is not possible. Further, where it has been tried, the core services approach has had limited impact in practice.[2]

In terms of the economic approaches discussed in the Toolkit, economic evaluation should be encouraged, but the focus here is generally on specific treatments or services. Thus, results from individual evaluations, at least for the purposes of priority setting, are best used within a broader framework or approach.[3] Another economic approach, which gained particular attention in the 1990s, is quality adjusted life years (QALY) league tables. This approach can be useful for setting priorities for new resources, but does not get at the notion of reallocating resources within a given budget. In addition, the QALY measure itself is quite narrow and does not capture non-health aspects of benefit.

Turning to PBMA, this approach incorporates the economic concepts of opportunity cost and the margin, and through the use of an advisory panel, examines how resources can be best allocated at various levels within health organisations.[4] The size and make-up of the panel will be dependent on the scope of the application, and evidence, in different forms (see Figure 5.1), can be drawn in to support the decision making process. PBMA is pragmatic in that when evidence is available and locally relevant, it can be used, but when it is not, greater reliance can be placed on the "expertise" of those on the advisory panel.[5] The added-value of PBMA, particularly in comparison to historical allocation processes, is that decisions are explicitly based on pre-defined criteria, both costs and benefits of treatment options are weighed at the margin, and investment and disinvestment decisions are considered in tandem.

In terms of the criteria, or principles, on which priority setting will be based, the key here is for these to be locally relevant and explicitly stated. These criteria may reflect the values of the organisation, the healthcare system, or more broadly, society at large. The issue is whose values count and how will those values be obtained. If a societal perspective is to be taken, members of the public can take a consultative role,[6] by providing input into criteria development. Decision makers can then make specific service provision decisions based on these criteria. As such activity requires additional resources, it may be that health organisations would rather develop the decision making criteria without broader consultation. Both approaches have pros and cons, but being explicit about what the criteria are and how they are to be developed will likely mitigate most problems.

Process evaluation

While PBMA provides the "nuts and bolts" for setting priorities, and in the end any number of outputs, including resource reallocation within a given budget can arise, focusing only on the outputs is inadequate. This is because it is important to also weigh out whether the process itself, irrespective of allocation recommendations, was fair and transparent.[7] One framework which has gained some attention in recent years is Accountability for Reasonableness. This framework enables the priority setting process that is applied in a given organisation to be evaluated against four ethical conditions. Conducting such an evaluation can thus provide important insight into how the priority setting process itself can be improved. This evaluation can take place through one-on-one interviews or focus group work with a broad range of stakeholders impacted through a given organisation's priority setting endeavours. A secondary benefit to conducting this type of evaluation, and revising the process accordingly, is that key stakeholders are much more likely to buy-in to a process that has been shown to be inherently "fair".

The challenges

In the second half of the Toolkit, a number of potential challenges were examined in some detail. For example, it is the case that data are required to carry out priority setting activity, and further, that such activity will take time. Part of the challenge of data is in populating a programme budget. The need for programme budgeting has also been called into question in the past. As well, it is the case that obtaining resource releases can be very difficult, particularly when incentives for change, such as fiscal pressure and information, are not present. Further, assessing the benefit of services can also be difficult, particularly when setting priorities across broad service areas. What information is relevant to obtain from the public, and how this is best captured, is another issue which requires due consideration when setting healthcare priorities. Importantly, all of these challenges can be overcome, and methods for this have been outlined in the Toolkit.

Moving forward hinges on what may well be the most challenging aspect of setting priorities in health care, that being organisational behaviour. Using data, finding time, releasing resources, mapping expenditure, capturing benefit and involving the public are all shaped by the organisational context and interpersonal interactions of the various stakeholders. In considering the barriers and facilitators to a priority setting process, as depicted in Figure 6.3, decision makers need to think about whether the right factors are in play in their organisation to embark on a process for setting priorities that is both explicit and informed. It is likely that personal and organisational incentives will assist in fostering an environment in which resource reallocation becomes part of routine planning, and various stakeholders, including physicians, become directly involved. What has been done in the Toolkit is to set out the parameters and present a reasonable way forward for priority setting, but enacting change and following-through on recommendations ultimately relies upon those who are charged with making the difficult decisions.

Recommendations

The economic concepts and methods outlined in the Toolkit are hopefully of value for managers and clinicians, in any type of healthcare system, who are seeking to identify how best to allocate available resources. It should be emphasised that organisations will likely be best served by conducting priority setting activity on an ongoing basis, and that it is only over time that measurable gains to population health can reasonably be expected. As such, monitoring and evaluation of priority setting decisions is paramount. Further, if there is a realisation, at some point in the future, that less than optimal choices were made, resources can always be reallocated elsewhere. Entrenchment of services has to become a way of the past in order to move to a place where resources are allocated in as best a manner as is possible. Sole reliance on new resources is problematic; the solution, at least in part, is in resource *re*allocation. Through the application of the concepts presented in the Toolkit, it is thought that direct input from academics in priority setting processes in health organisations could be minimised.

Waiting for perfect evidence or the very best approach will serve neither today's nor tomorrow's purposes for priority setting. The key recommendation here is to get on with the task of setting priorities in an explicit manner, noting that transaction costs may arise and mistakes will be made. It is well established that in competitive or entrepreneurial businesses, if you are not moving forward, you are in fact moving backward. To assist moving forward, it may be that health organisations would find it useful to develop a "priority setting team", which could be reassigned from current tasks, to carry out the processes outlined in this Toolkit.

Such a team should have clear links to the finance department (but generally should not be finance-department driven) and include or overlap with areas charged with programme evaluation. Further, it would be well served to have literature review and other research skills. Most importantly, the team leader, or project manager must be a champion and believer of the end objective. Ideally, the team would be "non-vested", and could thus serve as neutral entities when guiding priority setting activity. To help to ensure that the team does not get embroiled in organisational politics, reporting lines and placement within the structure of the organisation would need to be carefully considered. The priority setting team could also provide education on the economics behind priority setting, and might be expected to map out medium range plans for systematic roll out of a PBMA-like approach for priority setting both within and across programme areas. In the end, however, it is the decision makers themselves who ultimately must buy in to, and take responsibility for, allocation decisions.

Tying it all together

Referring to Figure 13.1, one could think of PBMA as the core package, around which various aspects of priority setting are based. If PBMA is to be successful, it must be conducted effectively, drawing on methodological lessons learned, as per Box 5.1 and Table 7.2. However, the PBMA process also needs to be set within the organisational context in which it is being applied, thus various barriers and facilitators to conducting explicit priority setting, and following-through on stated recommendations, as per Figure 6.3, must be given consideration. One vehicle for change, as used in the macro PBMA example provided in Chapter 7, is participatory action research, which has at its very centre the engagement of stakeholders and enacting of new processes to move an organisation towards its underlying aims. As part of engaging stakeholders and rewarding practice, incentives will likely be required, and in moving forward with change, education for the different actors will be key.

In addition, as is also highlighted in Figure 13.1, in order to support the priority setting activity, evidence on both costs and benefits is required, noting that evidence can come in various forms, and in some cases, greater reliance can be placed upon the opinions of those on the advisory panel. As well, community input may also be desired, through the development of the criteria on which decision making processes will be based, and potentially through eliciting preferences for health states. Any process should also seek to engage physicians and other clinical staff in some manner. Finally, if evaluation of the process is to be undertaken, the Accountability for Reasonableness framework can aid in determining if the process was intrinsically fair, and may inform re-working of the process or underlying principles over time. In the end, all of this might not be far off from current practice, but what Figure 13.1, and the Toolkit as a whole, does

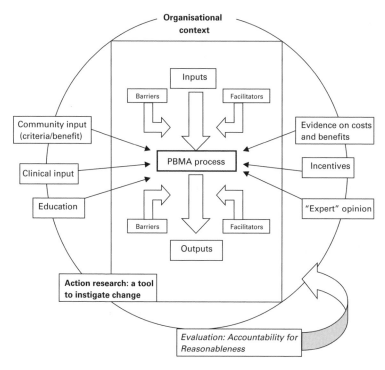

Figure 13.1 Depiction of aspects of priority setting

is to formalise the priority setting process, drawing attention to a set of tools to foster moving forwards and helping to ensure that the process is conducted in a transparent and explicit manner.

Further endeavours

While the Toolkit has outlined progression in the science and art of priority setting, it is clear that this is not an exact science, and uncertainties still exist. An important area for future research is to examine a broader sample of health organisations which have used PBMA in order to explore in greater detail the longer term (health) outcomes resulting from decisions made, and to identify further specific determinants for successful implementation of this approach. With such work, it would be important to examine factors such as the size of the health organisation, the employment of a health economist, and the familiarity with or prior use of economic evaluations. As well, issues pertaining to the organisational structure and informal managerial processes could be captured. Ideally, a construct of detailed points to consider when embarking on priority setting exercises would be developed and added to those already outlined in Figure 6.3.

In addition, in order to facilitate both further research in priority setting and practical application, collaboration with organisational behaviourists would likely be of great value. Managers, clinicians and health economists may not possess the change management skills required to foster widespread uptake of an explicit approach to priority setting, or the skills to ensure follow-through on recommendations. Important collaborations could also be struck with ethicists and other health services researchers who could bring added rigour both to criteria development, based on principles important to the broader community, and further, to process evaluation.

One key area that is impacted by the behaviour of the organisation, in terms of knowledge and available expertise, is measuring benefit. Further research is also required in determining how best to assess outcomes, particularly across service areas. Economic techniques such as willingness to pay and discrete choice experiments hold some promise but whether these approaches will have merit in practice, and whether they can be fully incorporated into an approach like PBMA, require further investigation. Finally, also in terms of organisational behaviour, more work is required in examining relationships – the importance of trust between stakeholders and collaboration across managerial and clinical boundaries is clear. How to foster such trust and collaboration needs further study.

Conclusion

Recognition that claims on resources will always outstrip resource availability in health care indicates a need to set priorities. Introducing an "economic way of thinking" within health organisations, through an approach like PBMA, should serve to aid decision makers in making difficult choices.

Decision makers may find it useful to take a pragmatic approach when assessing competing claims on limited resources, in that relevant evidence from the literature and elsewhere can be married with local data and expert opinion to make decisions. These decisions should be made at the margin, so that shifts in resource use will be examined and acted upon if benefit overall will be improved. Thinking in these terms can move a health organisation or specific programme area towards better meeting their pre-defined objectives, whether those objectives are related to efficiency or equity or both.

What we have done in this book is to show how an economic approach can be applied and embedded in day to day management practice. The approach outlined is pragmatic, widely used, sustainable, and brings a range of benefits to the organisation beyond the direct impacts on resource use and outcomes from decisions made. Using the economic approach presented here allows various claims on limited healthcare resources to be treated equally and to be given due process, enhancing the accountability, efficiency and equity of organisations that adopt it.

References

1 Culyer AJ. Equity – some theory and its policy implications. *J Med Ethics* 2001;**27**:275–83.
2 Maynard A, Bloor K. *Our Certain Fate: Rationing in Health Care.* London: Office of Health Economics, 1998.
3 Mitton C, Jarrell J. Economic evaluation in gynecology and obstetrics: principles and practice. *Can J Obstet Gynecol* 2003;**25**:219–23.
4 Peacock S. *An Evaluation of Program Budgeting and Marginal Analysis Applied in South Australian Hospitals.* Melbourne: Centre for Health Program Evaluation, Monash University, 1998.
5 Cohen D. Marginal analysis in practice: an alternative to needs assessment for contracting health care. *BMJ* 1994;**309**:781–5.
6 Litva A, Coast J, Donovan J *et al.* "The public is too subjective": public involvement at different levels of health-care decision making. *Soc Sci Med* 2002;**54**:1825–37.
7 Singer P, Martin D, Giacomini M, Purdy L. Priority setting for new technologies in medicine: qualitative case study. *BMJ* 2000;**321**:1316–18.

Index

Page numbers in **bold** text refer to figures in the text; those in *italics* refer to tables or boxed material